HEALTHY GUT HEALTHY HAIR

DECODING GUT BRAIN HAIR AXIS

DR. SUNIL MISHRA

Made with ♥ on the Notion Press Platform
www.notionpress.com

Contents

Acknowledgements

For

My parents, who teach me.
Dr. Rachita Dhurat, who guides me.
My wife and kids Dr Minal Mishra, Vedant and Adhyan, who inspire me.

Introduction

The Gut-Brain-Hair Connection
Unlocking the Secrets to Healthier Hair and a Happier You

What if I told you that the secret to healthy, luscious hair isn't hiding in your bathroom cabinet, but in a place far less glamorous, your gut? Yes, your gut, that hardworking digestive powerhouse you probably don't think about until it's making you uncomfortable, holds the key to more than just your digestion. In fact, the health of your gut directly influences the health of your hair, your brain, and pretty much everything else going on inside your body.

Welcome to the world of the gut-brain-hair axis a fascinating, intricate relationship between your digestive system, your mental state, and your hair growth. It's a connection that modern medicine is only just beginning to fully understand, but it's one that has the potential to transform the way you approach your health and your hair care for good.

You see, great hair isn't just about what you put on your head. It's about what's happening inside your body. Your hair is like the ultimate report card for your internal health: if things are going well on the inside, your hair will reflect it shiny, strong, and growing. But if something's off, whether it's stress, a gut imbalance, or poor nutrient absorption, your hair will sound the alarm. It might get thin, brittle, or even start falling out. And as anyone who's ever had a bad hair day can tell you, when your hair isn't thriving, it affects your confidence, your mood, and, let's face it, your whole outlook on life.

This book is your roadmap to stronger hair and a healthier you, but it's not going to tell you to spend hundreds of dollars on fancy shampoos or hair vitamins. Instead, it's going to take you on a journey deep inside your body, where the real work happens. We'll explore the role of gut health, dive into the fascinating connection between your brain and your hair, and uncover simple, sustainable lifestyle changes that can revolutionize your hair from the inside out.

Along the way, you'll learn about:

The microbiome: The trillions of bacteria in your gut that influence everything from your digestion to your mood and, yes, your hair growth.

Stress and cortisol: How stress hormones can wreak havoc on your hair and how you can manage them for a healthier, happier scalp.

Probiotics and prebiotics: How feeding your gut's good bacteria can supercharge your hair health.

Holistic health practices: From meditation to yoga to adaptogenic herbs, you'll discover how ancient wellness wisdom can support modern hair growth.

Practical tips: Easy, science-backed changes you can make to your daily routine that will benefit not just your hair but your overall health and well-being.

But don't worry this book isn't just a dry, medical lecture. It's written with a dose of humor, because let's face it: if we're going to talk about hair loss, gut bacteria, and meditation, we might as well have some fun with it! By the end of this book, you'll be armed with the knowledge to take control of your health, reduce stress, balance your gut, and grow the kind of hair that makes people stop and ask, "What's your secret?"

This isn't just another book about hair care it's about transforming the way you think about health and beauty from the inside out. While this book offers science-backed insights, it is not a substitute for medical advice. Always consult your doctor before starting any new health care or hair care regimen.

Ready to embark on the journey to better hair and a healthier, happier you?

Let's dive in!

CHAPTER ONE

THE GUT-BRAIN-HAIR TRIO

Now that you have bought this book and have shown interest in knowing about the association of Gut-Brain-Hair-Axis, let's start the journey without any delay. Picture this: you're at a concert hall, the lights dim, and suddenly, an orchestra explodes into action. Every instrument the violins, cellos, flutes, and trumpets blends together in perfect harmony, filling the room with sound so breathtaking it makes you forget that you're sitting in uncomfortable, overpriced seats. Now imagine your body as that orchestra. And the main performers? Your gut, your brain, and... your hair.

"Wait, what? Hair? What's it doing in this concert?" You might be thinking, "I get the gut it's busy dealing with that extra slice of pizza I regret eating. And the brain? Sure, it keeps me from texting my ex at 2 a.m. But what on earth does hair have to do with anything?"

Stick with me. Like a virtuoso triangle player in the background of a symphony, your hair is more important than you think. If any part of this trio gut, brain, or hair falls out of sync, the whole performance can quickly turn into a chaotic mess. Let's explore how these three unexpected buddies are connected and why they need to get along for you to stay healthy, and yes, to keep your luscious locks growing.

The Gut: More Than Just the Cheeseburger Digestor

Let's start with the gut. It's often misunderstood as just a boring, behind-the-scenes digestive worker, quietly handling your questionable food choices (looking at you, two-day-old samosa and pizza). But your gut is actually the Beyoncé of your body powerful, versatile, and capable of stealing the show. It's home to trillions of microorganisms, a lively, microscopic metropolis known as the gut microbiome.

Imagine it as Mumbai City in there microbes hustling, making deals, trying not to get hit by taxis, and keeping the whole operation running smoothly. These tiny citizens are responsible for digesting food, absorbing nutrients, producing essential vitamins, and even influencing your mood. Yes, they're multitaskers. Your gut is like the world's busiest CEO, managing your immune system, hormones, and even the condition of your skin. If it ever got a LinkedIn page, it'd make us all look lazy.

But what does any of this have to do with hair? Well, hair doesn't just magically grow because you decided to use expensive shampoo. The nutrients your hair needs to flourish biotin, zinc, iron, and vitamins D and E all come from the food you eat. But if your gut isn't breaking down and absorbing these nutrients properly, it's like throwing fertilizer on a sidewalk and expecting flowers to grow. Spoiler: *they won't.*

And let's talk about when things go wrong in this microscopic city. If your gut falls into chaos maybe because of stress, antibiotics, or that "all-pizza" diet you tried your microbiome gets thrown off balance. This leads to gut dysbiosis, the microbial equivalent of a Mumbai local train delay. Everything gets clogged up, toxic byproducts leak out, and the immune system freaks out. The result? Inflammation city and your hair follicles are some of the first citizens to feel the heat. Hair thinning, shedding, and breakage all follow, like bad backup singers ruining your perfect Beyoncé gut solo.

Gut Dysbiosis: Chaos in the City

When your gut is in turmoil, it affects your entire body. Think of gut dysbiosis as having the trash collectors in your city go on strike. All those nutrients you're supposed to absorb for hair growth? They're stuck in a traffic jam of chaos, and your immune system responds by lighting everything on fire in a very inflammatory way. Hair follicles, being the sensitive souls they are, start to shut down, taking refuge in the telogen (resting) phase, where they basically say, "I'm out, call me when this mess is over."

The hair's growth cycle is highly vulnerable to stress and inflammation. So if your gut is in disarray, expect your hair to start acting like a diva in a soap opera fainting, disappearing, and not showing up when you need it most. So the next time you notice extra hair in the shower drain, don't immediately blame your conditioner. Take a look at what's happening in your gut.

The Brain: More Than a Stress Machine

Ah, the brain. It's like that know-it-all conductor in our body orchestra, waving its baton and shouting, "More cortisol!" at the slightest hint of stress. You see, the gut and brain are constantly chatting like two old ladies gossiping on the phone. This long-distance conversation happens through the gut-brain axis, a direct communication line that uses the vagus nerve as its telephone wire.

And here's the kicker: the brain often decides to send stress signals down to the gut, which, of course, messes up digestion, leads to more inflammation, and you guessed, it affects your hair. Ever noticed more hair shedding during finals week or after a breakup? That's your brain throwing your gut off balance, which then throws your hair follicles into chaos.

Cortisol: The Ultimate Hair Saboteur

Let's talk about cortisol, the stress hormone that's as popular as a terrible office manager. When you're stressed, cortisol rises, and the body essentially goes into survival mode. This is great if you're being chased by a bear, but not so great if you're just sitting at your desk binge-watching shows. Cortisol tells your body, "Listen, we don't have time for non-essential tasks right now, like growing hair! We need to focus on keeping you alive."

In this stressed state, your body puts hair growth on the back burner. Your hair follicles shift into the resting phase, causing more shedding than usual. It's like your body saying, "No time for beauty right now, we've got a crisis here!" Chronic stress can even lead to conditions like telogen effluvium, where massive amounts of hair suddenly jump ship.

Hair: The Drama Queen

Let's not forget our star of the show: your hair. Hair is basically the canary in the coal mine of your health. When something's wrong internally, it's one of the first places you'll see it. Stress, poor diet, inflammation, or hormone imbalances? Your hair will let you know by shedding, thinning, or just generally looking like it's had enough of your nonsense.

Think of your hair as that one friend who's always super honest with you. You know, the one who tells you, "You've been stress-eating pizza again, haven't you?" and, "Maybe you should've gone to bed at a reasonable hour instead of doom-scrolling." It's a physical indicator of what's happening inside your body.

Hair grows in cycles: anagen (growth phase), catagen (transition phase), and telogen (resting phase). When everything's working well, your hair stays in the anagen phase longer, meaning it grows lush and thick. But when your gut or brain falls out of balance, more hair moves into the telogen phase, and you'll notice it shedding faster than the plot of a reality TV show.

Hair: The Canary of Health

So, what's the lesson here? Your hair is the visual, external marker of your internal health. If your gut is throwing a tantrum, if your brain is screaming, "More cortisol, more stress!", your hair will be the one silently shedding in the corner, trying to tell you that things aren't okay.

Next time you're freaking out about hair loss, don't just reach for the most expensive hair serum you can find. Ask yourself: how's my gut doing? Am I stressed out of my mind? Am I getting the nutrients I need? Because your hair is only as healthy as the systems that support it.

Conclusion: The Trio in Harmony

The gut-brain-hair axis is a delicate symphony, and when it plays in harmony, everything sounds (and looks) great. Your gut microbiome keeps things in balance, your brain stays chill, and your hair grows like a field of daisies. But throw just one of them off, and you're dealing with a chaotic, hair-shedding cacophony.

In the coming chapters, we'll dive deeper into this intricate relationship, revealing practical steps you can take to restore balance to the gut-brain-hair axis. We'll explore gut health hacks, brain-boosting strategies, and hair care secrets that will have you rocking your healthiest mane yet. So buckle up we're just getting started in this wild, fascinating world of the gut-brain-hair connection!

CHAPTER TWO

Microbial Maestros

Let's take a trip, not to Paris or Bali, but deep inside your gut trust me, it's more exciting than it sounds. Imagine your gut as a bustling metropolis, where tiny microorganisms (we'll call them gut bugs) are the industrious citizens. These gut bugs don't wear suits or carry briefcases, but they are every bit as important as CEOs running billion-dollar companies. Except, instead of worrying about stock prices, they're more concerned with keeping you alive, happy, and surprisingly... keeping your hair on your head.

Yep, your hair's fate isn't just in the hands of your shampoo or your stylist. Turns out, your gut microbiome the bustling ecosystem of bacteria, fungi, and viruses that live inside your intestines plays a major role in your hair's health. Who knew that your next bad hair day might actually be the result of a tiny riot happening in your gut?

In this chapter, we're going to dive deep into this microbial metropolis, understanding why the health of your gut could be the secret to flaunting luscious locks. It's time to give these gut bugs the recognition they deserve!

The Gut Microbiome: A Quick Overview (AKA, the "Gut Bug" Society)

Your gut is home to trillions of microorganisms. To give you an idea of the numbers: if gut bugs were concertgoers, they could fill every stadium on Earth... 10 times over. In fact, there are more of them than there are human cells in your body. They are the unsung heroes of your inner ecosystem, doing everything from helping you digest food to regulating your mood. But here's the kicker they're also working behind the scenes, quietly ensuring that your hair doesn't fall out by the handful every time you comb it.

You see, this microbial society isn't just there for digestion. It has major influence over your immune system, hormone production, and, as we're about to find out, the health of your hair. When the gut bugs are thriving, it's like a well-run city. But when they start slacking off whether because you've been living off fast food or because stress has turned you into a ball of cortisol it's chaos, and your hair follicles are among the first to notice.

The Gut-Brain-Hair Axis: A Comedy of Connections

Remember that quirky friend in Chapter 1 the brain? Well, your gut and brain are in constant communication. It's like they're texting each other all day long about what's going on. This is called the gut-brain axis, and it's not just small talk. They're actually gossiping about your stress levels, your nutrient intake, and yes, even how well your hair is doing. Imagine the gut texting the brain: "Hey, things are inflamed down here, let the follicles know!" The brain replies, "Got it. More cortisol inbound! Tell the hair to brace for some shedding."

So, when the gut-brain conversation is full of compliments (good food, low stress), your hair thrives. But when it's full of complaints (stress, processed foods, or antibiotics), your hair goes into survival mode, and survival mode doesn't include looking fabulous.

Gut Health and Hair Growth: A Tale of Nutrient Delivery Gone Wrong

Let's break down how your gut actually affects your hair. Your hair has a life cycle it grows, rests, and eventually falls out, kind of like that deadbeat roommate who never pays rent but takes up all the space. Most of your hair should ideally be in the anagen (growth) phase, which can last for years. This is when your hair is growing long, strong, and shiny, just the way you like it.

But, like a high-maintenance friend, hair demands attention and resources. It doesn't just grow because you want it to, it needs a steady supply of nutrients. And where do those nutrients come from? You guessed it: your gut. The microbiome breaks down food and helps your body absorb the vitamins and minerals your hair is dying for literally. It's like the UPS delivery service for your follicles.

Nutrients like biotin, vitamin B12, iron, and zinc are non-negotiables if you want healthy hair. Biotin, for instance, is a VIP nutrient for hair growth, and it's produced by your gut bugs. If the delivery service gets held up (thanks to gut issues like dysbiosis), your hair ends up with a "Sorry, We Missed You" notice instead of the nutrition it needs.

When the gut isn't in top form maybe because you've been stress-eating an entire pizza or because you forgot that vegetables exist it struggles to absorb the nutrients your hair needs. Your follicles, being dramatic little things, throw a fit. They start shedding more hair, growing weaker strands, and giving off that dry, brittle look that no amount of expensive serum can fix.

Gut Dysbiosis: The Microbial Version of a Traffic Jam

Gut dysbiosis is what happens when the bad bacteria in your gut stage a coup and overthrow the good bacteria. Dysbiosis throws everything out of balance: your digestion, your immune system, and yes, even your hair growth.

Inflammation becomes rampant when your gut is in disarray. Chronic inflammation is like an annoying house guest who refuses to leave, causing damage everywhere it goes including your hair follicles. Inflammation disrupts the normal hair growth cycle, shortening the anagen phase and pushing more hair into the telogen (resting) phase, where it will eventually fall out. It's like hitting the pause button on hair growth while your body fights an internal battle.

Hair Loss: The Gut's Protest March

Gut dysbiosis can even lead to more extreme hair loss conditions like alopecia areata, where your immune system mistakenly attacks your hair follicles. And guess what? Scientists are discovering that people with these hair loss conditions often have higher levels of gut inflammation. So, while you're busy blaming your genetics or your shampoo, your gut is quietly trying to tell you, "Hey, I'm the problem here."

A disrupted gut microbiome can also lead to leaky gut syndrome (yes, that's a real thing). Leaky gut is what happens when the lining of your intestines gets damaged, allowing toxins and bacteria to escape into your bloodstream. It's like your gut walls are letting in the riffraff, leading to even more inflammation and triggering autoimmune reactions including ones that target your hair.

Good Bacteria, Good Hair

On the flip side, a healthy gut means happy hair. A balanced microbiome is like a well-run government it makes sure everything gets done smoothly and on time. The good bacteria in your gut produce short-chain fatty acids (SCFAs) that keep inflammation under control and support immune function, which is critical for keeping your hair follicles in top shape.

In fact, the more diverse your gut microbiome, the better your hair health. Studies have shown that people with stronger, thicker hair tend to have more diverse microbiomes. It's like having a versatile workforce of gut bugs that can handle any crisis, ensuring your body (and your hair) stays in balance.

Probiotics and Hair: The VIPs of Gut Health

Now enter probiotics, the A-list celebrities of the gut health world. Probiotics are live microorganisms that help repopulate your gut with beneficial bacteria. You can find them in fermented foods like yogurt, kimchi, sauerkraut, and kombucha, or in supplements. They're like the superheroes your gut needs to restore balance and keep everything in check.

Adding probiotics to your diet helps reduce inflammation, improve nutrient absorption, and support your immune system all things that contribute to healthier hair. Specific strains like Lactobacillus and Bifidobacterium have even been shown to lower inflammation, which is great news for your follicles.

Prebiotics: The Gut Bug Fuel

Of course, probiotics need to eat too! That's where prebiotics come in. Prebiotics are the food that good bacteria thrive on, and they come in the form of fiber found in foods like garlic, onions, asparagus, and bananas. If probiotics are the VIPs, then prebiotics are the catering team that keeps them going.

Feeding your gut bacteria with prebiotics helps ensure that they can perform their many important tasks including keeping your hair healthy. Without the right fuel, even the best probiotics won't be able to work their magic.

Gut Health and Scalp Drama: The Plot Thickens

And the drama doesn't stop with your hair strands. A compromised gut can also mess with your scalp. Ever wondered why you're suddenly battling dandruff or experiencing scalp irritation? Your gut bugs might be throwing shade at your scalp. Conditions like dandruff, seborrheic dermatitis, psoriasis, and eczema are often linked to gut imbalances.

For instance, an overgrowth of Malassezia (a fungus that lives on your scalp) can be triggered by gut dysbiosis, particularly if you've got a yeast overgrowth happening internally (looking at you, Candida). When your gut is out of whack, your immune system struggles to keep things balanced, which can lead to scalp flare-ups and even hair thinning.

Conclusion: Keep the Symphony Playing

Your gut microbiome isn't just a random collection of microorganisms hanging out in your intestines. It's the conductor of a complex symphony that keeps your body and your hair in harmony. When your gut is balanced, you absorb nutrients like a pro, reduce inflammation, and keep your hair follicles happy. But when dysbiosis strikes, it's like the orchestra hits a sour note, and your hair is the first to suffer.

So, if you're serious about growing that Pinterest-worthy mane, it's time to start focusing on your gut. Load up on prebiotics and probiotics, limit the processed junk, and maybe stop stress-bingeing on ice cream during Netflix marathons. By treating your gut with the respect it deserves, you'll be giving your hair the best possible chance to shine literally.

Now, who's ready to let their gut bugs take center stage for some well-orchestrated hair health?

In the next chapter, we'll dive into another important topic: the enteric nervous system, the gut feeling also known as the second brain. We'll explore how this gut-based brain influences hair growth and why gut health is so deeply connected to your mental and emotional well-being. Get ready for a journey into the gut-brain-hair connection like never before!

CHAPTER THREE

Gut Feelings, Your "Second Brain"

You've probably heard of the brain that squishy, walnut-shaped thing in your skull responsible for all your brilliant ideas, questionable life decisions, and occasional obsessions with late-night snacks. But did you know that your gut has a brain too? Yes, your enteric nervous system often called the "second brain" resides in your digestive tract, and it's a big deal when it comes to everything from digestion to mood regulation to, you guessed it, hair growth.

Now, before you start imagining your intestines holding mini TED talks or solving algebra problems, let me clarify: the second brain isn't writing poetry or pondering the mysteries of the universe. But it does play a vital role in managing your overall health, influencing everything from your immune system to your stress levels both of which are intimately connected to your luscious (or not-so-luscious) locks.

In this chapter, we're diving deep into your gut's brain, exploring how it controls more than just digestion, and why having a happy gut is one of the most powerful things you can do for your hair. Plus, we'll discuss how to give your second brain the TLC it needs to keep those strands strong and flowing.

Meet Your Second Brain: The Enteric Nervous System

So, what exactly is this enteric nervous system (ENS)? Essentially, it's a vast network of neurons (the same kind you have in your actual brain) that reside in the lining of your gut. The ENS is so extensive that it contains about 100 million neurons that's more than your spinal cord! If that's not impressive enough, consider this: the ENS operates independently of your brain. That's right your gut has its own decision-making power when it comes to digestion.

This doesn't mean it's plotting world domination (although it does seem to plot cravings for pizza and chocolate at the worst times), but the ENS does manage digestion without needing to consult your head brain. It's like your gut has its own personal assistant, handling all the mundane tasks so your brain can focus on more important things like binging your favorite Netflix series.

The Gut-Brain Axis: Important Long-Distance Relationship in Your Life

Even though your gut's brain operates independently, it still communicates with your head brain on a regular basis, like two co-workers who text each other constantly even after work hours. This ongoing dialogue happens through the gut-brain axis, a two-way communication system that uses nerves, hormones, and chemical messengers to keep your brain and gut in sync. The biggest star of this show is the vagus nerve, a sort of superhighway that connects your gut to your brain.

Now, here's where things get interesting. This connection doesn't just regulate digestion, it affects stress, mood, and even your hair growth. When your gut is out of balance, it sends stress signals to your brain, and when your brain is stressed, it sends signals to your gut. This back-and-forth stress train is not only terrible for your mental health but also for your hair. Cortisol, the stress hormone, loves nothing more than to ruin a good hair day.

Stress, Hair, and Your Gut's Brain: The Triangular Tussle

Let's talk about stress. Stress is like the frenemy of life it pretends to help in emergency situations but more often than not, it overstays its welcome and wreaks havoc on everything, including your hair. When you're stressed, your central nervous system (brain and spinal cord) goes into fight-or-flight mode, which is great if you're being chased by a lion but less useful when you're late for a meeting or watching your favorite team lose.

In fight-or-flight mode, your body directs energy away from "non-essential functions" like digestion and hair growth to focus on survival. Unfortunately, your hair doesn't get the memo that the "danger" is just your phone not working during a conference call, so it stops growing and sometimes starts falling out. And where is all this stress heading? To your gut. The stress signals sent by your brain end up in your gut, where they disrupt the microbiome, leading to gut imbalances that can further mess with your hair.

Yes, your gut brain and head brain are both guilty parties when it comes to stress-induced hair loss, making them the dynamic duo you didn't want but are stuck with.

The Enteric Nervous System's Role in Hair Growth

The enteric nervous system doesn't just sit around managing digestion and getting frazzled by stress. It also plays a key role in regulating inflammation and nutrient absorption, two things that are directly related to your hair's health. Let's break it down:

1. Inflammation Control

We've talked about inflammation being a hair villain before, but your second brain is like the unsung superhero trying to fight back. The ENS helps regulate the gut's immune system, working to keep inflammation in check. When your gut is healthy, it's like a well-oiled machine that produces anti-inflammatory compounds, keeping everything calm and collected including your hair follicles.

But when things go haywire (due to poor diet, stress, or gut imbalances), the ENS can't regulate inflammation properly, leading to systemic inflammation that reaches all the way to your scalp. This can trigger hair loss conditions like telogen effluvium or alopecia areata (fancy terms for "your hair is making a mass exit").

2. Nutrient Absorption

The ENS also controls how well your gut absorbs nutrients, think of it as the quality control manager at a factory. It oversees the absorption of vitamins, minerals, and proteins, all of which are crucial for hair growth. Nutrients like biotin, vitamin D, zinc, and omega-3 fatty acids are the building blocks of strong, shiny hair.

But when the ENS is stressed or dysfunctional, nutrient absorption goes out the window. It's like trying to fill a leaky bucket no matter how much you pour in, you're not getting enough. Without proper nutrient absorption, your hair becomes malnourished, brittle, and prone to breakage.

The Gut Feeling: Trusting Your Second Brain's Signals

You know that feeling when your stomach flips before an important meeting or you get a "gut feeling" about something? That's your second brain talking, and you should probably listen. Gut feelings aren't just something made up by romantics they're real. Your gut brain communicates with your head brain to regulate mood, make decisions, and even let you know when you're stressed. So, when your gut is out of balance, you'll feel it not only in your body but also in your mood.

Why is this important for your hair? Because stress and anxiety whether it's from a gut imbalance or an external issue trigger hair loss. Your hair is essentially the sensitive flower of your body, wilting at the first sign of trouble. If your gut is sending stress signals to your brain, your hair is one of the first things to suffer.

How to Keep Your Second Brain Happy (and Your Hair Fabulous)

Now that we know your second brain plays a huge role in how your hair looks and feels, it's time to talk about how to keep it happy. The good news? It's not as hard as it sounds. Here's how to make sure your gut brain is cool, calm, and collected (and, by extension, your hair is fabulous):

1. Eat to Fuel Your Gut's Brain

Your second brain thrives on nutrient-rich, gut-friendly foods. Think of it like this: your gut brain doesn't want pizza and soda any more than your actual brain wants constant reality TV reruns. Give it the good stuff:

Fiber-rich foods: Vegetables, whole grains, legumes, and fruits help keep your gut bacteria in balance.

Fermented foods: Add some yogurt, sauerkraut, or kimchi to your diet to boost the beneficial bacteria in your gut and keep your ENS running smoothly.

Omega-3s: Salmon, flaxseeds, and walnuts are packed with omega-3 fatty acids, which reduce inflammation and support gut health.

2. Manage Stress (or Try to)

Easier said than done, I know. But managing stress is crucial for keeping your second brain from sending panic signals to your head brain (and vice versa). Incorporating stress-relief techniques like yoga, meditation, or just a daily morning walk can work wonders for calming both your brains. Think of it as pressing the reset button for your body and mind plus, your hair won't be under constant attack.

3. Get Moving

Exercise isn't just for keeping your muscles in shape it also helps keep your gut in tip-top condition. When you move, your gut moves too, promoting better digestion and reducing inflammation. Plus, exercise releases endorphins, which counteract stress hormones and make both your brains happy.

4. Sleep Like a Pro

Sleep is when your body repairs itself, including your gut. Your ENS loves a good night's sleep it uses that downtime to reset, reduce inflammation, and keep your gut bacteria in balance. Aim for 6-8 hours of quality sleep each night to keep your second brain and hair in optimal condition.

5. Supplement Smartly

If your diet alone isn't enough to keep your gut happy, certain supplements can help. Probiotics, for example, introduce beneficial bacteria into your system, while digestive enzymes can support your gut in breaking down food. Other options include magnesium (great for calming stress) and omega-3 supplements for inflammation.

Conclusion: Let Your Second Brain Lead the Way

Your enteric nervous system might not be giving TED talks or solving world peace, but it's doing a pretty great job of keeping your body running. When it's in balance, you feel good, your digestion works well, and your hair thrives. But when it's stressed, inflamed, or out of whack, your hair pays the price. By supporting your gut brain with the right food, stress management, and healthy habits, you can keep both your brains happy and rock some seriously great hair in the process.

Next up, we'll delve deeper into the relationship between brain-gut connection, stress and cortisol everyone's favorite stress hormone and how they wreak havoc on your hair.

CHAPTER FOUR

How Your Mind and Gut Influence Hair

You've heard of bad hair days, right? But what if I told you that your brain and gut are planning most of those without even consulting you? That's right, the drama that unfolds on your scalp could be a direct result of the gossip happening between your brain and gut. Today, we dive into this bizarre love triangle the brain-gut-hair connection where your stress and anxiety can wreak havoc on your hairline. So buckle up! It's time to meet the real culprits behind your thinning locks: your brain's overactive stress hormones and your gut's flare-up of rebellion.

The Brain-Gut Axis: The Gossip Hotline You Never Knew You Had

Let me introduce you once again to the brain-gut axis. It's a constant conversation between two of your body's major players: your brain (a bit of a control freak) and your gut (the moody artist type). They're in constant communication, sending each other messages through a hotline known as the vagus nerve. Think of it like a gossip line where your brain spills the tea to your gut about stress and anxiety, and the gut gossips back about how it's upset because you ate that questionable burger last night.

Ever felt nervous and suddenly had to rush to the bathroom? That's your gut receiving a 100 call from your brain. Or maybe you've had stomach problems when you're stressed at work. Your gut and brain don't just chat about digestion; they also discuss important matters like inflammation, immunity, and yes hair growth. It's the kind of gossip that ends with you shedding more than just tears.

How Stress and Anxiety Hijack Your Gut and Your Hair

Stress is that one unwelcome guest who comes to your party and eats all the chips. You thought it would be a quick visit, but then they stay too long, mess up the furniture, and make everything worse. When stress overstays its welcome, your brain releases cortisol the body's go-to "stress hormone." In small doses, cortisol is like a superhero, helping you react to danger. But when stress becomes chronic, cortisol turns into a villain, disrupting everything, including your hair's life cycle.

Chronic stress puts your body in survival mode. Think of it like the Titanic everything unnecessary (like hair growth) gets thrown overboard to keep the essential systems (your heart, lungs, and brain) afloat. Meanwhile, your gut goes into panic mode, throwing its hands up and saying, "I can't handle this!" Cue gut dysbiosis (aka, when your gut bacteria party too hard and chaos ensues), nutrient absorption grinds to a halt, and inflammation skyrockets.

Cortisol: The Sneaky Hair Assassin

Meet cortisol, the sneaky ninja of hair loss. Under normal conditions, your hair enjoys a luxurious stay in the anagen phase (the growth phase) for a few years. But cortisol, being the stress-loving troublemaker it is, shortens this phase and shoves your hair into the telogen phase (resting phase). Your hair basically gets furloughed and eventually "quits," falling out more than your patience when your Wi-Fi goes down.

This condition, where stress accelerates hair shedding, is called telogen effluvium. If your shower drain is starting to look like it needs a toupee, cortisol could be the culprit. What's worse? Telogen effluvium can last for months if you don't deal with your stress. Think of it as a long, passive-aggressive breakup with your hair, one strand at a time.

Anxiety's Role: When Your Brain Just Won't Chill

Now, let's talk about anxiety. If stress is the drama queen, anxiety is the relentless paparazzi, always there, never letting your nervous system take a break. Anxiety keeps your body in a constant fight-or-flight mode, where everything's on high alert, even when you're just trying to pick out a cereal in the grocery store.

This endless state of tension throws your digestion off the rails. Your gut motility (the movement of food through your digestive system) slows down or speeds up unpredictably, making you feel bloated, constipated, or both. And when your gut can't digest properly, your hair is one of the first to suffer from nutrient deprivation. It's like trying to water your plants when your garden hose is kinked nothing is getting through!

But wait, there's more. Anxiety often messes with your eating habits. Some people stress-eat like they're preparing for hibernation, while others lose their appetite altogether. Either way, it's bad news for your hair. Poor eating habits lead to vitamin and mineral deficiencies, and your hair is left starving for nutrients like biotin, iron, and zinc the Holy Trinity of hair health.

The Gut as the Real Mood Boss

You think your mood is all about what's happening in your brain? Not so fast. Your gut is the backstage manager, producing 90% of the body's serotonin, a neurotransmitter that plays a big role in keeping you feeling happy and calm. When your gut is out of whack, serotonin production tanks, and guess what? Your mood follows. Cue anxiety, stress, and you guessed it, more hair loss.

So, in this tangled mess, it's your gut saying, "If you're not going to take care of me, I'll make sure your hairline pays for it." And let's face it, no one wants to be in that situation.

Stress Management: Because Your Hair Deserves Better

Here's the good news: you can actually manage your stress and anxiety. No, seriously. There are proven ways to tell your brain and gut to sit down, be humble, and let your hair grow in peace. Here's how:

1. Mindfulness Meditation: Because Cortisol Needs a Timeout

Take 10 minutes of early morning mindfulness meditation. I know, sitting still sounds counterproductive, but hear me out. Mindfulness meditation helps you focus on the present, letting go of the endless "what ifs" that feed your anxiety. Studies show that it reduces cortisol levels and improves your gut health, allowing your hair follicles to get back to their full-time job: growing.

2. Deep Breathing: Like CPR for Your Gut and Brain

Deep breathing exercises, like 4-7-8 breathing (inhale for 4 seconds, hold for 7, exhale for 8), can activate your parasympathetic nervous system the one responsible for calming everything down. When this system kicks in, your gut says, "Finally, I can digest in peace!" and your brain chills out. It's like sending both of them on a much-needed vacation, which means fewer cortisol spikes and more time for your hair to stay in the growth phase.

3. Regular Exercise: But Don't Go Overboard

Exercise is the ultimate stress-buster. It lowers cortisol, boosts your mood with endorphins, and gets your blood (and nutrients) flowing to your hair follicles. But beware: over-exercising can have the opposite effect, raising cortisol levels and causing stress-induced hair loss. So, keep it balanced aim for moderate exercise like 45 mins of walking, yoga, or cycling in morning. You're not training for the Olympics here; your hair needs you to be a calm, collected human.

4. Probiotics: The Hair-Growth Sidekick

Who knew that probiotics could help your hair grow? Certain strains like Lactobacillus rhamnosus and Bifidobacterium longum have been shown to reduce anxiety and cortisol levels by supporting the gut-brain axis. They're like the peacekeepers in this whole saga, helping your gut get its groove back. Incorporate probiotic-rich foods like yogurt, kefir, sauerkraut, and kimchi into your diet or go for a quality supplement if fermented foods aren't your thing.

5. Sleep Hygiene: Because Even Your Hair Needs a Good Night Rest

If you're not sleeping well, you're missing out on prime hair-growing time. Poor sleep raises cortisol levels, disrupts digestion, and leaves you feeling more frazzled than before. Aim for 6-8 hours of solid, uninterrupted sleep. Avoid caffeine, turn off your screens at least an hour before bed, and try a relaxing bedtime routine. Trust me, your hair will thank you for it.

Conclusion: A Brain, A Gut, and A Hairline Walk Into A Bar...

The moral of this story? When your brain, gut, and hair team up, they can either form a powerhouse of wellness or a tag team of stress-induced chaos. Chronic stress and anxiety can tip this trio out of balance, leading to gut dysbiosis, nutrient deficiencies, and, ultimately, hair loss. But with the right strategies like stress management, probiotics, and mindfulness you can restore peace to the brain-gut axis and give your hair the love it deserves.

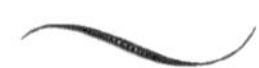

CHAPTER FIVE

CORTISOL, CHAOS, AND HAIR LOSS

Ah, stress. We all know it, we all hate it, and if stress were a person, it would be the one that shows up uninvited to every party, ruins your night, and somehow manages to eat all the chips without bringing any of its own. It's that relentless part of life that affects everything your mood, your health, and yes, your hair. And behind this stress-induced hair catastrophe is a sneaky hormone named cortisol, just sitting there like a villain twirling its metaphorical mustache.

In this chapter, we're diving deep into the vicious cycle of stress, cortisol, and hair loss because nothing says "fun weekend read" like exploring how stress messes with your hair. But don't worry, it's not all doom and gloom. By the end of this chapter, you'll know exactly how to outsmart cortisol, manage stress, and give your hair a fighting chance against life's constant plot twists.

Cortisol: The Stress Hormone with an Agenda

Before we get into how cortisol sabotages your hair, let's get to know this hormone a little better. Cortisol is the body's main stress hormone. Produced by the adrenal glands (those little triangle-shaped things on top of your kidneys), cortisol is part of your body's "fight-or-flight" response. Back in the day when stress meant running away from saber-toothed tigers cortisol was incredibly useful. It gave you a burst of energy, heightened your senses, and shut down non-essential systems (like digestion and hair growth) so you could focus on survival.

But here's the thing: in today's world, we're not exactly running from wild beasts. Instead, our stress comes from bills, work deadlines, parking tickets, and endless Zoom meetings that could've been emails. Yet, your body still reacts to these stresses like it's facing a life-or-death situation, pumping out cortisol like it's going out of style.

And while cortisol was once your knight in shining armor, in the modern world, it's become more like that friend who only brings drama constant, exhausting drama. When cortisol levels remain high for too long, it wreaks havoc on your body. Your immune system gets compromised, your digestion goes haywire, and cue the dramatic music your hair starts to fall out.

How Stress and Cortisol Tag-Team Your Hair

Stress and cortisol are like the dynamic duo you didn't ask for, teaming up to pull a fast one on your hair. Here's how it goes down:

**1. Cortisol Throws Your Hair into the Resting Phase
(Because It Needs a Nap)**

Your hair grows in cycles: the anagen phase (growth phase), the catagen phase (transition phase), and the telogen phase (resting phase). Ideally, your hair spends most of its time in the anagen phase, growing long and strong like a fairytale princess locked in a tower. But when cortisol crashes the party, it cuts the anagen phase short and sends a bunch of your hair into the telogen phase.

Why? Because cortisol thinks you're in danger and your body has bigger things to worry about than luscious locks. "Survival first, hair later," says cortisol, shoving your poor hair into the backseat. Unfortunately, hair in the telogen phase eventually falls out and that's when you start noticing more strands clogging your shower drain, as if they're staging a dramatic exit from your scalp.

2. Inflammation: Cortisol's Sidekick

As if shoving your hair into early retirement wasn't bad enough, cortisol also stirs up inflammation throughout your body. We've talked about inflammation before (and how it's basically the enemy of everything good in life), but here's the refresher: when inflammation hits, it affects your hair follicles by making them inflamed, irritated, and, well, uncooperative.

Think of it this way: your hair follicles are like tiny factories working to produce strong, healthy strands of hair. But when cortisol triggers inflammation, it's like someone called a strike at the hair follicle factory. Suddenly, nothing gets done, production halts, and your hair follicles decide they're just going to hang out in "do nothing" mode for a while. Great, right?

3. Nutrient Blockade: The Ultimate Sabotage

Cortisol is like that annoying person who steals all the Wi-Fi bandwidth at the coffee shop you're just trying to get things done, but now everything is slowed to a crawl. In the same way, cortisol disrupts nutrient absorption in your gut, preventing key vitamins and minerals like biotin, iron, and vitamin D from reaching your hair follicles. Without these nutrients, your hair can't grow properly, and even the healthiest strands can become weak and brittle.

Your gut, already struggling under the weight of stress and inflammation, can't function optimally, and your hair suffers as a result. So even if you're eating all the right foods (cue spinach smoothies and cucumber beetroot salads), your body is too stressed to fully absorb the nutrients you need for hair growth. Cortisol has essentially installed a toll booth in your gut, charging you extra just to get the nutrients to your hair. Rude.

Stress-Induced Hair Loss: Three Types Yoyou need to Know About

By now, you're probably thinking, "OK, cortisol is the worst. But how does stress actually show up on my scalp?" Well, stress-induced hair loss comes in a few different forms. Here are the three major players:

1. Telogen Effluvium: The Hair Shed of Doom

Telogen effluvium is the most common form of stress-induced hair loss. Remember how cortisol throws your hair into the telogen phase like it's handing out free vacation tickets? Telogen effluvium occurs when too much hair enters the resting phase all at once. The result? A dramatic increase in hair shedding, like you've suddenly become the star of a slow-motion shampoo commercial except instead of tossing around a full head of hair, you're watching it fall to the floor.

The good news? Telogen effluvium is usually temporary. Once the stress subsides, your hair can start growing back. The bad news? It can take several months for your hair to fully recover, which is why dealing with stress ASAP is key.

2. Alopecia Areata: The Patchy Betrayal

If telogen effluvium is the stress-induced shedding, alopecia areata is the ultimate betrayal. In this autoimmune condition, your immune system confused and cranky, thanks to chronic stress starts attacking your own hair follicles. This leads to patchy bald spots, which can range from small areas to large, more noticeable patches. It's as if your hair is playing hide-and-seek, except you're not really in on the game.

Alopecia areata can be triggered by a combination of stress, genetics, and other factors, and in severe cases, it can lead to complete hair loss. While it's often reversible, it's definitely one of the more frustrating forms of stress-induced hair loss.

3. Trichotillomania: The Stress Pull

Some people react to stress by stress-eating, some by stress-shopping, and some by stress-pulling... their hair. Trichotillomania is a condition where people compulsively pull out their own hair, often without realizing it. It's linked to anxiety and stress, and over time, it can lead to noticeable hair thinning or bald patches. This form of hair loss is less about cortisol and more about the direct toll stress takes on behavior.

Breaking the Vicious Cycle:
How to Outsmart Stress and Save Your Hair

Here's the thing: stress is inevitable. Bills will come, work will get busy, and parking tickets will still make you curse the heavens. But while you can't eliminate stress entirely, you can manage it and reduce its impact on your body (and your hair).

1. Get Moving

I know, I know exercise is the solution to everything. But seriously, physical activity is one of the best ways to reduce cortisol levels and release those feel-good endorphins that make your brain feel like it just got a warm hug. Whether it's yoga, running, dancing, or just walking the dog, regular exercise helps keep cortisol in check and prevents it from running the show.

2. Embrace Your Inner Zen Master

You don't need to become a full-on meditation guru, but finding ways to de-stress on a daily basis is crucial for controlling cortisol. Try deep breathing exercises, meditation apps, or even just taking five minutes a day to sit in silence and let your brain chill out. Bonus: meditation doesn't just lower cortisol it can also improve your mood, sleep, and overall health.

3. Sleep Like It's Your Job

When it comes to managing stress and hair health, sleep is like that one friend who actually shows up on time and brings snacks to the party. Getting enough quality sleep helps your body repair and recover from the stresses of the day, keeping cortisol levels in check and giving your hair the chance to grow in peace. Aim for 6-8 hours of sleep per night (and no, doomscrolling in bed doesn't count as "winding down").

4. Eat the Good Stuff

Your diet plays a huge role in how well your body handles stress. Foods rich in omega-3 fatty acids (like salmon and walnuts), magnesium (think spinach and almonds), and B-vitamins (hello, leafy greens) are all great for reducing cortisol and inflammation. Now you can literally eat your way to less stress.

5. Consider Adaptogens (AKA Nature's Chill Pills)

If stress is a constant companion in your life, you might want to look into adaptogens herbs that help your body adapt to stress. No, this isn't the name of a new hipster band or the next superhero franchise it's a group of herbs that help your body adapt to stress (hence the name, clever right?). Adaptogens are like your body's chill-out squad, working behind the scenes to make sure you don't lose your mind every time something goes wrong, which, as we know, directly impacts your gut and, of course, your hair.

In the world of holistic health, adaptogens are the MVPs, calming down your adrenal glands and keeping your cortisol levels from turning you into a stressed-out mess. And since we've already established that cortisol is basically the hair villain of this story, adaptogens can play a starring role in giving your hair a fighting chance.

Top Adaptogens for Hair Health

Ashwagandha: This ancient herb from India has been used in Ayurvedic medicine for centuries, and it's the granddaddy of adaptogens. Ashwagandha helps lower cortisol levels, reducing stress and inflammation, and improving both your gut and hair. Basically, it's the herb you want in your corner when life gets overwhelming (which, let's be honest, is pretty much all the time).

Rhodiola: If you're the kind of person who operates at 100 mph and feels burned out by 10 AM, rhodiola is your herb. It's great for fighting fatigue, lowering stress, and boosting your mood. With less stress and better mental clarity, your gut calms down, your body absorbs more nutrients, and your hair says "thank you" by stopping the mass exodus from your scalp.

Holy Basil: Holy basil isn't just regular basil that went to church, it's an adaptogenic herb used to calm stress and support gut health. It's also anti-inflammatory and helps reduce oxidative stress, which is the fancy way of saying it's the body's fire extinguisher. When your body's stress response cools off, your hair follicles can focus on growing instead of panicking.

6. Aromatherapy: Smelling Good Can Actually Help Your Hair Grow

Aromatherapy might seem like something you'd find in a spa gift basket, but it's actually a powerful tool for stress management, gut health, and surprise! hair growth. Certain essential oils have been shown to improve circulation, reduce stress, and even stimulate hair follicles. And the best part? You get to smell amazing while you do it.

Best Essential Oils for Hair Growth

Rosemary oil: If there's one essential oil that deserves a medal for hair growth, it's rosemary oil. Studies have shown that rosemary oil can be effective for promoting hair growth. It works by improving blood circulation to the scalp, which helps hair follicles get the nutrients they need to thrive.

Lavender oil: Lavender oil isn't just for helping you fall asleep it's also a powerful anti-inflammatory that soothes the scalp and reduces stress. Since stress is one of the main culprits behind hair loss, adding a few drops of lavender oil to your daily routine is basically like giving your hair a day at the spa.

Peppermint oil: Want to wake up your scalp? Peppermint oil gives a refreshing tingle that not only smells good but also increases circulation and promotes hair growth. Plus, your scalp will feel minty fresh, which is always a bonus.

To get the most out of these oils, mix a few drops with a carrier oil (like coconut or jojoba oil) and massage it into your scalp. You'll be boosting circulation, calming your nervous system, and giving your hair follicles the wake-up call they've been waiting for.

7. Acupuncture: Sometimes You Need to Get to the Point (Literally)

Acupuncture may sound a little terrifying at first (because, you know, needles), but this ancient practice is a staple of Traditional Chinese Medicine and has been used for thousands of years to treat all kinds of ailments including stress, inflammation, and hair loss. Plus, after you get over the idea of being a human pincushion, acupuncture is actually quite relaxing kind of like napping in a serene room, but with extra health benefits.

How Acupuncture Helps Your Hair

Acupuncture works by stimulating energy flow (or Qi) throughout your body. When energy gets blocked, it can lead to inflammation, stress, and health issues (including hair loss). By inserting super-thin needles into specific points on the body, acupuncture helps clear up these blockages and gets your body back in balance. And guess what? When your body is balanced, your gut is happy, and when your gut is happy, your hair follows suit.

In modern medical terms, acupuncture promotes blood circulation, which helps deliver more oxygen and nutrients to your hair follicles. It also lowers stress hormones, so your body can stop freaking out and start focusing on hair growth again. Plus, it's a great excuse to tell your friends that your wellness routine is "on point." (Sorry, had to.)

Conclusion: The Stress-Hair Balance

While stress might be a fact of life, losing your hair doesn't have to be. By managing stress, keeping cortisol in check, and taking care of your body with healthy habits, you can break the vicious cycle of stress-induced hair loss and keep your mane looking its best even when life throws you the occasional curveball (or parking ticket).

So, let's give cortisol the boot, calm that anxious brain, and tell your gut bugs to get back to work. The result? Happy hair that stays firmly on your head, and a lot less shedding drama. Stay tuned for the next chapter, where we tackle inflammation the other silent troublemaker in the gut-brain-hair saga

CHAPTER SIX

INFLAMMATION, THE HIDDEN THREAT TO YOUR HAIR

Imagine your body is a peaceful village, where your gut, brain, and hair live in harmony. But lurking in the shadows, there's an arsonist who just can't leave well enough alone its name? Inflammation. At first, it's helpful, like the fire department rushing in to deal with an emergency. But when it sticks around too long, it turns into that annoying neighbor who keeps setting off fireworks at 2 a.m. Chronic inflammation is the sneaky villain that quietly sabotages everything, including your precious hair.

In this chapter, we're going to reveal the devious ways inflammation messes with your body, and more importantly, how it's throwing your hair follicles into a tailspin. But don't worry, we'll also arm you with strategies to douse this inflammatory fire before it burns down your hair growth goals.

What Is Inflammation? The Good, the Bad, and the Ugly

Inflammation gets a bad rap, but it's actually a crucial part of your body's defense system. Imagine you cut yourself slicing an apple (because let's face it, who hasn't?). Your body immediately sends out the inflammation squad immune cells, proteins, and chemicals to deal with the damage, neutralize any potential invaders, and start the healing process. This type of acute inflammation is like a superhero swooping in to save the day.

But sometimes, the inflammation squad doesn't get the memo that the crisis is over, and they decide to hang around like uninvited guests who just won't leave. This is chronic inflammation, and instead of saving the day, it causes collateral damage, breaking down healthy tissues, organs, and yes, your hair. Chronic inflammation is like trying to put out a fire by throwing gasoline on it. And your hair follicles are not fans of this approach.

The Hair Follicle vs. Inflammation: A Lose-Lose Battle

Your hair follicles, those tiny factories responsible for growing your hair, are incredibly sensitive to inflammation. When your body is dealing with chronic inflammation, it disrupts the hair growth cycle. Instead of chilling in the anagen phase (the growth phase) for years, your hair gets pushed into the telogen phase (resting phase) way too early, like being kicked out of the club before the party even starts.

This leads to telogen effluvium, a condition where way too much of your hair is chilling in the resting phase and then decides to jump ship. Over time, chronic inflammation can also trigger more severe forms of hair loss, like alopecia areata, where your immune system basically declares war on your hair follicles. Bad times, indeed.

The Usual Suspects: Inflammatory Conditions Targeting Hair

Let's meet the lineup of inflammatory conditions that are particularly good at wrecking your hair:

1. Alopecia Areata

This autoimmune disorder has your immune system mistakenly targeting your hair follicles, leading to patches of hair falling out faster than a bad toupee in a windstorm. The exact cause isn't fully understood, but chronic inflammation, often linked to gut health issues, leading to auto immune condition is thought to play a role in sending your follicles into hiding.

2. Seborrheic Dermatitis

Imagine your scalp is a flaky croissant, seborrheic dermatitis causes inflammation, itching, and flaking on your scalp, disrupting the hair follicles in the process. It's often linked to an overgrowth of yeast (not the sourdough kind, sadly) and can be worsened by gut dysbiosis.

3. Psoriasis

This fiery condition causes red, scaly patches to pop up on your skin and scalp, leading to hair shedding. Psoriasis is an autoimmune condition tied closely to systemic inflammation and gut health, making your hair the unwilling victim of an internal battlefield.

The Gut: Your Body's Anti-Inflammatory Headquarters

Here's where things get really interesting: your gut isn't just in charge of digesting last night's burrito it's the command center for inflammation in your body. When your gut is happy, it produces anti-inflammatory compounds like short-chain fatty acids (SCFAs) that keep inflammation levels in check. It's like having a team of firefighters constantly on standby, ready to put out any sparks before they turn into a wildfire.

But if your gut is in trouble say, from a poor diet, chronic stress, or illness the barrier that protects your gut from the rest of your body gets compromised. This leads to leaky gut syndrome, where toxins, bacteria, and undigested food particles escape into the bloodstream. Picture your gut as a leaky ship, with water pouring in and causing inflammation to flood your entire system, including your hair follicles. Your immune system freaks out and starts attacking anything in sight hello, inflamed hair follicles!

Inflammatory Foods: The Fire Starters in Your Diet

Now let's talk about the obvious culprits inflammatory foods. Certain foods are like gasoline for the inflammation fire, and if you're regularly consuming them, your hair is going to feel the heat. Here's what to watch out for:

Processed foods: Full of refined sugars, unhealthy fats, and artificial chemicals, these foods are inflammation central. They might be convenient, but your hair will pay the price.

Sugar: Think of sugar as inflammation's best friend. It spikes blood glucose levels, causing your body to release inflammatory markers. Plus, it's addictive, so good luck cutting it out.

Trans fats: Found in fried foods and baked goods, these are like tiny inflammation grenades going off inside your body.

Alcohol: Excessive drinking can damage your gut lining, leading to you guessed it more inflammation. So, if you're constantly raising a glass, your follicles might be raising a white flag.

Anti-Inflammatory Foods: The Heroes Your Hair Deserves

On the flip side, an anti-inflammatory diet can be your secret weapon for luscious locks. Here's what to load up on to keep inflammation at bay:

Omega-3 fatty acids: These are like the fire extinguishers of inflammation. Found in fatty fish like salmon, chia seeds, and flaxseeds, omega-3s can cool down inflammation and keep your hair growing strong.

Leafy greens: Spinach, kale, and Swiss chard are packed with antioxidants and nutrients that fight inflammation, making them the hair heroes you never knew you needed.

Berries: These little powerhouses (blueberries, strawberries, raspberries) are rich in antioxidants that help neutralize free radicals, reducing oxidative stress and inflammation.

Turmeric: This golden spice contains curcumin, a super-powerful anti-inflammatory compound. Think of it as inflammation's kryptonite. Bonus points if you combine it with black pepper to boost absorption.

Green tea: Filled with antioxidants called catechins, green tea has anti-inflammatory effects that can benefit your gut, brain, and hair. So sip away your follicles will thank you.

Lifestyle Changes: Calm the Inflammatory Storm

Sure, diet's a big part of the equation, but lifestyle also plays a crucial role in taming the inflammatory fire.

Some habits to keep your inflammation and your hair under control:

1. Regular Exercise

Exercise lowers inflammation by promoting the release of anti-inflammatory cytokines. But don't go overboard too much intense exercise can actually trigger inflammation, so balance is key. Think of early morning yoga, walking, or a light jog, not a boot camp where you're crying into your protein shake.

2. Stress Management

Chronic stress is like throwing logs on the inflammatory fire. The more stressed you are, the more cortisol floods your system, causing inflammation to skyrocket. Find ways to relax whether it's meditation, deep breathing and your body will respond by lowering inflammation levels.

3. Quality Sleep

You've heard it before, but it's worth repeating: sleep is crucial for keeping inflammation in check. Aim for 6-8 hours of quality sleep a night to allow your body time to repair and restore. Plus, your hair grows more while you sleep so it's a win-win!

Supplements to Keep Inflammation in Check

If diet and lifestyle aren't quite enough, there are supplements that can help you tackle chronic inflammation head-on:

Omega-3 supplements: If you're not a fan of fish, take a fish oil or flaxseed oil supplement to get your dose of inflammation-fighting omega-3s.

Turmeric (Curcumin): A curcumin supplement can work wonders in reducing inflammation, especially when combined with black pepper to enhance absorption.

Probiotics: Restore balance to your gut microbiome with a high-quality probiotic supplement, preferably one containing Lactobacillus and Bifidobacterium strains.

Vitamin D: Many people are deficient in vitamin D, especially in the colder months. This powerhouse nutrient helps regulate the immune system and inflammation, so consider a supplement if you're running low.

Conclusion: Time to Fire the Saboteur

Inflammation might be the silent saboteur of your hair, but it doesn't have to win. By addressing the root causes of chronic inflammation whether they stem from your diet, stress, or gut imbalances you can stop unnecessary hair shedding in its tracks. So fuel your body with anti-inflammatory foods, chill out on the processed junk, manage your stress, and get some solid sleep. Your gut, brain, and hair will all thank you.

In the next chapter, we'll dive even deeper into the world of toxins and detoxification because every good mission requires a clean escape. Stay tuned, agent!

CHAPTER SEVEN

TOXINS, DETOX, AND HAIR REVIVAL

Cue dramatic detective music. The scene: your once-thriving scalp is looking a little... suspicious. Hair has started vanishing in mysterious ways more in the shower drain, more on your brush, less on your head. You're no stranger to the usual suspects: stress, genetics, maybe some bad hair days. But what if I told you there's a secret villain at play, operating from the shadows? The villain's name: Toxins. And it's time to solve the case.

Join me, Detective Detox, as we embark on a thrilling investigation into how toxins are silently sabotaging your luscious locks and how we can bring the culprit to justice through the power of detoxification. Cue magnifying glass zoom on hair follicles.

Understanding Toxins: The Shadowy Figures in the Background

We live in a world crawling with toxic agents chemicals, pollutants, plastics, and more, all waiting for the right moment to strike. These silent intruders are everywhere, hiding in your air, food, water, and even that seemingly innocent shampoo bottle. They've infiltrated your system and are wreaking havoc on your hair. But what exactly are these toxins, and why are they so interested in your scalp?

Toxins are like the sneaky crooks in a crime drama they slip into your body and start messing with everything from hormone regulation to cellular health, leaving chaos in their wake. These shady characters can come from outside (like air pollution, pesticides, heavy metals) or even inside (the byproducts of your body's own metabolism or gut bacteria gone rogue). And once they start hanging around, they set off alarms in the form of inflammation, which you now know is terrible news for your hair.

The Suspects: Meet the Toxin Gang

- **Environmental Toxins:** These bad boys include air pollutants, pesticides, heavy metals like lead and mercury, and chemicals found in plastics (like BPA and phthalates). They sneak into your body through the air you breathe, the water you drink, and even the lotions you slather on your skin.
- **Endogenous Toxins:** These are the toxic byproducts your body naturally produces during normal metabolic processes. It's like your body's waste management system but if the garbage truck goes on strike, this trash builds up and creates a whole mess for your cells and your hair.
- **Endocrine Disruptors:** These sneaky chemicals target your hormones. Found in plastics, pesticides, and certain personal care products, they mimic or block hormones, leading to imbalances that can cause your hair to shed faster than a detective losing their cool in a high-stakes interrogation.
- **Pathogenic Toxins:** The shady dealers lurking in your gut. When your gut health is out of whack (say, due to gut dysbiosis), harmful bacteria and yeast like Candida can produce their own toxins, which then damage your gut lining and send inflammatory messages all over your body, including your scalp.

So now that we've identified the suspects, it's time to ask: how exactly do these toxins pull off their heist against your hair?

The Gut: The Mastermind Behind the Scenes

Welcome to HQ your gut. This is where the real investigation begins because the gut is critical to how toxins are managed in your body. It's like the security system of a high-end vault. If everything's working smoothly, toxins are kept out, neutralized, or escorted off the premises via your digestive system. But if your gut's compromised (think leaky gut,

gut dysbiosis, or a poor diet), it's like leaving the vault doors wide open for toxins to stroll right into your bloodstream and set off a chain reaction of damage.

A healthy gut does more than just digest your spinach salad. It acts as a barrier, keeping dangerous toxins out of the system while helping your body eliminate waste efficiently. But when the gut is weakened, toxins pass through, triggering inflammation and adding pressure on the liver, kidneys, and hair follicles. Now, your follicles are caught in the crossfire of this internal sabotage. The result? Your hair starts falling like evidence in a poorly planned crime scene cleanup.

The Liver: Your Detox Powerhouse (aka The Cleanup Crew)

Enter the liver, your body's #1 detox agent. It's like the forensics team, sweeping through the body to filter out toxins, break them down, and eliminate them. It's also tasked with handling some key players in the hair game: hormones like estrogen and testosterone. But when the liver is overworked whether from a poor diet, environmental pollutants, or hormone imbalances it gets sluggish. Imagine trying to mop up a crime scene with one hand tied behind your back. Not very effective.

A sluggish liver means toxins start building up in your body, leading to oxidative stress (a fancy way of saying your cells are getting wrecked) and inflammation. Both of these spell disaster for your hair follicles. The liver also manages hormone metabolism, so if it's not doing its job right, you could end up with conditions like estrogen dominance or elevated DHT levels both major suspects in the case of hair loss.

The Inflammatory Trail

Every good detective knows to follow the trail. And in this case, it leads us to one big clue: inflammation. Chronic exposure to toxins leads to long-term inflammation, which is like throwing a bomb into your hair's growth cycle. It damages hair follicles, messes with nutrient absorption, and cuts short the time your hair spends growing, causing it to fall out faster than you can say "detox."

The toxic villains are smart, though. They also cause gut issues that prevent your body from absorbing key hair-loving nutrients like biotin, zinc, and iron. Without these nutrients, your hair doesn't stand a chance thinning, breaking, and shedding are all inevitable. We need to stop this toxic chain of events before it's too late.

Supporting Detoxification: How to Turn the Case Around

Time to go from clue-finding to action! Here's your step-by-step detective work for supporting your body's natural detox processes and giving your hair the healthy environment it deserves:

1. Hydrate Like Your Hair Depends On It (Because It Does)

Water is your body's trusty sidekick in flushing out toxins. It helps your kidneys and liver work efficiently, keeping toxins from building up. Aim for at least 8 glasses a day, and throw in a squeeze of lemon for bonus detox points. Lemon is loaded with vitamin C and antioxidants, both of which are like reinforcements for your liver's detox team.

2. Eat Your Way to Victory: Foods That Detox and Defend

You need food that'll stand by your side, not sabotage your mission. Here are your hair health allies:

Cruciferous Vegetables: These include broccoli, Brussels sprouts, and cabbage. They contain sulforaphane, a compound that helps the liver detoxify and eliminates harmful substances.

Leafy Greens: Spinach, kale, and arugula are packed with chlorophyll, which binds to toxins and helps escort them out of the body.

Beets: These little red detectives support liver function and reduce oxidative stress. They also help boost bile production, which is key for flushing out toxins.

Garlic and Onions: These allium vegetables help neutralize heavy metals and support the liver's detox work.

Turmeric: The ultimate anti-inflammatory spice. Turmeric's secret weapon is curcumin, which reduces oxidative stress and promotes hair health.

3. Call in the Herbal Backups

Certain herbs act like the special agents in your detox team:
Milk Thistle: Protects and regenerates liver cells, ensuring that detoxification runs smoothly.
Dandelion Root: Stimulates bile production, helping the liver clear out toxins more efficiently.
Burdock Root: Cleanses the blood and supports liver function, all while improving circulation to your hair follicles.

4. Break a Sweat: The Sweaty Interrogation

Sweating is your body's built-in interrogation method getting toxins to sweat out their secrets. Whether you exercise or hit the sauna, sweating helps eliminate heavy metals and toxins stored in your fat cells. These saunas help detoxify at a deeper level, boosting circulation and supporting hair regeneration.

5. Reduce Exposure: Keep the Criminals Out

The best way to avoid a repeat crime? Limit your exposure to the toxin gang:
Ditch plastics (BPA, we're looking at you) and opt for glass containers.
Use natural, non-toxic personal care products. Skip the harsh chemicals in your shampoo, conditioner, and skincare.
Choose organic produce when possible to avoid pesticide exposure.
Filter your water to remove pollutants like chlorine, fluoride, and heavy metals.

Conclusion: Case Closed Toxins Busted, Hair Regained

With the clues uncovered, we've pieced together the mystery of hair loss: toxins. These hidden criminals have been silently infiltrating your body, messing with your hormones, inflaming your gut, and sabotaging your hair. But fear not, Detective Detox has shown you the way to bring them to justice!

By supporting your body's natural detox systems keeping your gut in check, hydrating, eating detox-friendly foods, sweating it out, and reducing exposure you'll give your hair the fighting chance it needs to recover, regenerate, and thrive.

In the next chapter, we'll tackle how hormones influence hair health and how gut health can help keep your hormonal balance in check. Get ready to dive into the world of estrogen, cortisol, and all the other key players that secretly run the show when it comes to hair growth!

CHAPTER EIGHT

Gut Health, Hormonal Harmony and Hair

Deep in the shadows of your body, there's an unseen but powerful force that can either make your hair flourish or abandon ship. No, this isn't a covert spy mission, but it might as well be. You've heard about "agents" in spy movies pulling the strings behind the scenes, right? In the case of your body, hormones are those secret agents, stealthily dictating everything from mood and metabolism to you guessed it hair growth. But like any good spy story, there's a twist: your gut is the headquarters of this covert operation. If your gut's on a mission gone wrong, it can set off a chain reaction that leaves your hair looking like it's been caught in an explosion.

So, buckle up, agent this mission takes us deep into the world of hormonal sabotage, gut intrigue, and the hair-raising (or hair-losing) results that come when things go awry.

Understanding Hormones and Hair Growth: The Secret Agents

Hormones, much like secret agents, are the ultimate multitaskers. They move silently through your bloodstream, delivering coded messages to your organs and tissues, telling them what to do and when to do it. And when it comes to your hair? Hormones hold all the power. They control whether your hair will be thick and strong or decide to take an early vacation off your scalp.

Here's your intel on the key hormonal agents influencing hair growth:

Estrogen and Progesterone: The James Bonds of hair. Estrogen keeps hair in the anagen (growth) phase longer, which is why women often enjoy luxuriously thick hair during pregnancy. Progesterone plays the role of a sidekick, balancing estrogen and keeping the scalp healthy.

Testosterone and DHT: These are the rogue agents. Dihydrotestosterone (DHT) is the evil twin of testosterone, a master villain that shrinks hair follicles and sends them into early retirement. DHT is the main culprit behind androgenetic alopecia, aka pattern baldness in both men and women.

Cortisol: Cortisol is the stress agent who's always freaking out and pulling the emergency brake on hair growth. Too much cortisol can shorten the hair's growth phase, pushing it straight into telogen effluvium where shedding becomes your new reality.

Thyroid Hormones: These are the logistics agents, managing your energy, metabolism, and you guessed it hair growth. If these agents are slacking, you'll notice your hair getting thinner, slower to grow, or just plain brittle.

Insulin: The double agent you didn't know was in the game. While it's best known for regulating blood sugar, insulin can also mess with hair by influencing other hormones, like testosterone. When insulin goes rogue (hello, insulin resistance), it can lead to hair loss, especially in women with conditions like PCOS.

The Gut-Hormone Connection: HQ's Got a Leak

In this operation, your gut is the HQ (Headquarters) for hormonal action. You see, the gut isn't just there to digest your food; it's also where hormones get broken down, metabolized, and either put to good use or kicked out of the body. If HQ is compromised due to dysbiosis, leaky gut, or other gut issues those hormones start going rogue. And when hormones are out of balance, your hair is often the first to feel the fallout.

Here's how the gut controls the hormone game:

Detoxification and Hormone Clearance: The gut is like the janitor for excess hormones. It helps remove used-up estrogen, cortisol, and other hormones from the body. But when the gut's out of order (maybe constipation's got the pipes clogged), those hormones get reabsorbed into the bloodstream, causing all sorts of chaos like estrogen dominance and hair loss.

Neurotransmitter Production: The gut is also a key player in making serotonin and dopamine, chemicals that keep your mood in check. Low serotonin means higher cortisol (hello, stress!) and more hair falling out faster than a spy can disappear into the night.

Regulation of Inflammation: Chronic inflammation is the mole in your system, quietly sabotaging your hormonal balance. If your gut is inflamed, it disrupts hormone production, leading to a hormonal cold war that could end with you shedding more hair than you'd like.

The Estrobolome: Hidden deep in your gut is the estrobolome, a group of bacteria tasked with managing estrogen levels. When this team is running smoothly, excess estrogen is broken down and cleared out. But if these bacteria are missing in action, estrogen starts throwing its weight around, causing estrogen dominance, which can lead to hair thinning and other issues like PCOS and endometriosis.

Estrogen: The Good Agent Gone Rogue

Estrogen is a powerful ally when it's on your side. It helps your hair stay in the anagen phase, allowing it to grow longer and thicker. That's why during pregnancy (when estrogen is through the roof), many women experience luscious, Disney-princess hair. But when estrogen levels drop like after childbirth it's as if the mission is over, and your hair starts evacuating the premises faster than you can say "postpartum hair loss."

On the flip side, when estrogen goes rogue and levels get too high (thanks to gut issues reabsorbing it), you end up with estrogen dominance. This imbalance can wreak havoc on your hair, causing it to thin or fall out entirely. Estrogen dominance is often linked to gut problems because, remember, HQ is in charge of eliminating excess estrogen. When it fails, your hair follicles feel the burn.

Testosterone and DHT: The Hair Saboteurs

Meet DHT, the secret double agent of the hair world. While testosterone has its fair share of influence, DHT is the real villain behind hair loss. It binds to hair follicles, shrinking them down until they're too small to produce decent hair (miniaturization of hair). In both men and women, high DHT levels are responsible for androgenetic alopecia (pattern baldness).

But how does the gut come into play? Glad you asked:

Insulin Resistance: When your gut is off balance, it can lead to insulin resistance, where your cells stop responding properly to insulin. This is common in conditions like PCOS, which often goes hand in hand with higher testosterone and DHT levels, leading to you guessed it hair loss.

Inflammation: Chronic inflammation promotes the conversion of testosterone into DHT, fueling the hair loss fire. So if your gut is inflamed, you've essentially hired DHT as the villain of your follicular film.

Gut Flora: Specific bacteria in the gut help metabolize hormones, including testosterone. When those bacteria go MIA, hormone levels rise, and your hair follicles shrink in fear.

Cortisol: The Stress-Hormone Snitch

Ah, cortisol, the ever-stressed secret agent who just can't keep it together. Normally, cortisol's job is to help you escape danger (like running from a lion or a bad haircut). But in today's world, we're constantly stressed, and cortisol levels stay elevated. This is bad news for your hair.

Prolonged high cortisol levels force hair follicles into the telogen phase prematurely, where they stop growing and start shedding. It's like cortisol is telling your hair, "We've got bigger problems than you right now!" Add in the fact that cortisol also contributes to leaky gut and inflammation, and you've got a recipe for hormonal imbalance and hair loss.

Thyroid: The Logistics Team That Can't Keep Up

Your thyroid is the logistics agent that oversees metabolism, energy, and yes hair growth. When the thyroid is slacking off, it leads to hypothyroidism, where everything, including hair growth, slows down. You'll notice your hair getting brittle, thinning, and breaking faster than cheap spy equipment.

But it gets worse: your gut is responsible for converting thyroid hormone T4 into its active form, T3, which directly influences hair growth. When the gut's compromised, this conversion process slows down, leaving you with all the signs of hypothyroidism without the official diagnosis. It's like trying to run a covert mission with no intel nothing works the way it should.

How to Balance Hormones for Hair Health: Operation Rescue

It's time to restore order and get your hair back on track. Here's the plan for balancing your hormones and saving your follicles from certain doom:

1. Support Gut Health

The gut is mission control for hormonal balance. Load up on probiotics (found in yogurt, sauerkraut, and kefir) and prebiotics (think garlic, onions, and asparagus) to keep your gut bacteria happy and efficient.

2. Eat for Hormone Balance

Focus on foods that help maintain hormonal harmony:
Healthy fats like omega-3s reduce inflammation and support hormone production.
Fiber helps eliminate excess estrogen, keeping estrogen dominance at bay.
Cruciferous vegetables like broccoli and Brussels sprouts contain DIM, which helps metabolize estrogen.

3. Manage Stress Like a Pro

Incorporate stress-relieving activities into your routine to keep cortisol under control think meditation, deep breathing, and exercise. This way, you'll prevent cortisol from calling the shots in your hair's growth cycle.

4. Nutrient Reinforcements

Make sure you're getting enough zinc, vitamin D, magnesium, and B-vitamins. These help regulate hormone production and give your hair the support it needs to thrive.

5. Get Some Sleep

Sleep is your secret weapon for resetting your hormonal balance. Aim for 6-8 hours of quality sleep, so your body has time to repair and regulate.

6. Avoid Endocrine Disruptors

Stay away from chemicals like phthalates and BPA (found in plastics and some personal care products) that mess with your hormones. Go natural where you can it'll keep your hormones happy and your hair happier.

Conclusion: Hormonal Harmony Is the Key to Hair Glory

Much like a well-planned spy mission, everything in your body is connected and when it comes to hair health, hormones are the ones pulling the strings. But remember, your gut is HQ, and if it's compromised, the whole mission goes sideways. By supporting your gut, managing stress, and keeping your hormones in check, you can restore harmony and bring your hair back from the brink.

Next up, we'll dig deeper into the role of diet and its impact on your hair health. It's time to learn how to build the perfect nutritional roadmap for strong, resilient hair that doesn't flinch at the first sign of stress!

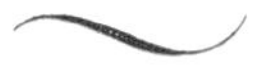

CHAPTER NINE

FEED YOUR HAIR FROM THE INSIDE OUT

Picture this: your body is like a hair salon, your gut is the shampoo girl, your brain is the stylist, and your hair... well, your hair is the picky customer. What your hair demands most? The finest nutrients delivered in the perfect balance. But if the shampoo girl (your gut) doesn't absorb the right nutrients or the stylist (your brain) gets too stressed out, the customer (your hair) storms out, leaving a trail of split ends, thinning strands, and shedding all over the floor. Let's dive into how your diet yes, the one that includes late-night snacks and questionable "superfood" trends plays a starring role in shaping your hair's destiny.

In this chapter, we're going to pull back the salon curtain and reveal the real secret to hair health: nutrition. We'll explore the exact nutrients your hair craves, how they get absorbed (or don't) in the gut, and what happens when your nutritional highways hit a traffic jam. Spoiler alert: those bad hair days might not be your shampoo's fault.

The Role of Nutrients in Hair Growth: Feed Me, Seymour!

Your hair is kind of like that demanding houseplant you keep forgetting to water. It needs constant nourishment to thrive because it's one of the fastest-growing tissues in your body (yep, hair is needy like that). Let's break down the VIP nutrients that make your hair grow and shine like a diva at a red carpet event.

1. Protein: The Building Blocks of Good Hair

Hair is basically a big ol' strand of keratin, a protein that gives it structure and strength. Without enough protein, your hair becomes weak, breaks easily, and looks like it's given up on life. You wouldn't build a house out of sand, so why would your hair want to grow without its essential protein?

2. Iron: The Oxygen Delivery Service

Iron is like the Uber driver for your hair it delivers oxygen to your follicles. No oxygen? No growth. When iron levels are low (thanks to deficiencies or poor diet), your body pulls a fast one and decides, "Hair can wait. Let's focus on keeping the heart and brain alive." The result? Your hair enters the resting phase and you start shedding like a golden retriever in summer.

3. Zinc: The Follicle Repairman

Zinc is the handyman of your hair world it's involved in cell growth and repair, making sure your follicles are in tip-top shape. A zinc deficiency leads to thinning hair and slow growth, like trying to fix a leaky faucet without a wrench. If you've got scalp issues, zinc's your guy.

4. Vitamin D: Sunshine for Your Hair

Your hair follicles are super hormonal no really, they love hormones. Vitamin D helps them create healthy follicles, which is essential if you're dreaming of thick, voluminous hair. Low levels of this sunny vitamin are linked to alopecia (hair loss), which explains why your hair might look a little sad in the winter months.

5. Omega-3 Fatty Acids: The Scalp Hydration Team

These healthy fats are the moisture kings of the hair world. They help reduce inflammation and keep your scalp hydrated. Think of them as the natural oils that keep your hair from turning into straw. Without omega-3s, your scalp dries up, flakes off, and your hair starts shedding like confetti at a parade.

6. B-Vitamins (Especially Biotin): The Energizer Bunnies

You've probably heard that biotin is the holy grail of hair growth, and there's some truth to that. B-vitamins, particularly biotin, help create red blood cells, which transport nutrients and oxygen to your scalp. Without them, your hair gets weaker and more prone to breaking. Fun fact: if you're low on biotin, your nails might also look like they've been through a blender.

Nutrient Absorption: The Gut as the Delivery Driver

So, you've been eating all the right foods, and yet your hair still looks like it's in a perpetual state of rebellion. What gives? The issue might be with your gut the real MVP when it comes to nutrient absorption. Your gut is like the delivery driver for all the nutrients your hair needs. If your gut's not working properly, those essential vitamins and minerals don't make it to their final destination: your hair follicles.

When you eat, your gut breaks food down into tiny nutrient pieces (think of it as your gut's version of IKEA flat-packing), which are absorbed through the intestinal walls into your bloodstream. From there, they're transported to your hair follicles. But if your gut's inflamed or struggling due to conditions like leaky gut or gut dysbiosis, it's like your delivery driver decided to skip your house. No nutrients, no hair growth.

Conditions like celiac disease, Crohn's disease, and even chronic constipation or diarrhea can mess with nutrient absorption. It's like the nutrients are stuck in a traffic jam, and your hair pays the price with thinning, shedding, and all-around sad vibes.

Nutrient Deficiencies and Hair Loss:
When Your Hair Waves the White Flag

Nutrient deficiencies don't just impact your energy levels and skin they're the reason why your hair might be staging a quiet protest. Here are the usual suspects and how to spot them:

1. Iron Deficiency (Anemia)

Iron deficiency is one of the biggest culprits behind hair loss, particularly in women. When iron's low, your body basically says, "Look, heart and brain get priority on oxygen. Hair follicles can take a pause." This leads to telogen effluvium, where your hair prematurely enters the resting phase and sheds more than normal.

2. Biotin Deficiency

Though rare, biotin deficiency can happen, especially if you have malabsorption issues or you're taking medications that interfere with biotin metabolism. If you notice brittle hair, thinning, or weird skin rashes, biotin could be the missing piece of your puzzle.

3. Zinc Deficiency

Lack of zinc can lead to slow hair growth, thinning, and scalp issues (hello, dandruff!). Without zinc, your follicles have a hard time regenerating, and your hair starts looking like it's been through a lot because it has.

4. Vitamin D Deficiency

Low vitamin D levels are linked to various types of hair loss, including androgenetic alopecia (pattern baldness) and alopecia areata (where you lose hair in patches). This sunshine vitamin is responsible for follicle regeneration, so if your levels are low, it's time to get outside or supplement.

5. Omega-3 Deficiency

Dry, brittle hair? Flaky scalp? You might be running low on omega-3s. These fatty acids keep your hair hydrated and your scalp nourished. Without them, your hair looks like it's been through a desert.

Foods for Healthy Hair: The Grocery List Your Hair Deserves

Now that you know what your hair needs, let's talk about where to get those nutrients. Here's the ultimate grocery list for hair that's strong, shiny, and ready to take on the world.

1. Eggs

Packed with protein and biotin, eggs are like the Swiss Army knife of hair health. They're also rich in zinc and selenium, making them a hair-boosting superfood. Plus, eggs are versatile you can eat them for breakfast, lunch, or dinner, or even slap one on your hair for a DIY mask.

2. Fatty Fish

Salmon, mackerel, and sardines are loaded with omega-3 fatty acids, which help reduce inflammation and nourish your scalp. They also contain vitamin D and protein, making them a triple threat for hair health.

3. Leafy Greens

Spinach, kale, and Swiss chard are packed with iron, vitamin C, and folate, all of which are crucial for oxygenating your hair follicles and promoting growth. Vitamin C also helps your body absorb iron more efficiently, making it the perfect partner in crime.

4. Nuts and Seeds

Almonds, walnuts, flaxseeds, and chia seeds are brimming with omega-3 fatty acids, zinc, and biotin. They're also great for snacking, so you can feel good about noshing on something that's fueling your hair growth.

5. Sweet Potatoes

These orange beauties are rich in beta-carotene, which your body converts into vitamin A. This promotes the production of sebum, your scalp's natural oil, keeping your hair hydrated and healthy. Think of sweet potatoes as hair moisturizers disguised as food.

6. Avocados

Loaded with vitamin E and healthy fats, avocados are like the hair superheroes you never knew you needed. Vitamin E acts as an antioxidant, protecting your hair from damage, while healthy fats nourish your scalp and follicles.

Hair Supplements: When Whole Foods Need a Little Backup

While it's always best to get your nutrients from food, sometimes life gets in the way (like when you've eaten pizza for three days straight). That's where supplements come in. Here's what you might consider adding to your routine:

1. Biotin

Although deficiencies are rare, biotin supplements are popular for promoting hair strength and growth. If your hair feels weak, this might help.

2. Iron

If you're dealing with low iron, a supplement can help reverse hair shedding. But be careful too much iron can actually be harmful, so get your levels checked before you pop a pill.

3. Vitamin D

For those of us living in gloomy climates, a vitamin D supplement is a must. It supports follicle health and helps keep hair in the growth phase.

4. Zinc

Zinc supplements can help if your levels are low, but don't overdo it too much zinc can mess with your body's balance of other minerals, like copper. Moderation is key!

5. Collagen

Collagen supplements are packed with amino acids that support not only hair but also skin and nails. Plus, collagen helps strengthen the gut lining, improving nutrient absorption for all-around health.

Crash Diets: The Fast Track to Hair Loss

Look, I get it. Crash diets promise the world: fast weight loss, glowing skin, eternal happiness. But here's the truth your hair hates them. When you drastically cut calories, your body goes into survival mode. It prioritizes essential functions (like keeping your heart pumping) over non-essential processes like hair growth. The result? Telogen effluvium aka stress-induced hair shedding.

So, if you're thinking about going on a cabbage soup cleanse or something equally tragic, please reconsider. Healthy, sustained weight loss is the only way to ensure your hair doesn't jump ship along with those extra pounds.

Conclusion: Fueling Your Hair from the Inside Out

The secret to healthy, vibrant hair isn't in a bottle of shampoo, it's in your diet. By focusing on nutrient-dense, whole foods and supporting your gut health, you can give your hair the nourishment it craves. Sure, the occasional supplement can help, but nothing beats a well-rounded, balanced diet when it comes to growing strong, resilient hair.

Next up in our investigation, we're going deep into the world of gut dysbiosis, a major suspect in the case of hair sabotage. Stay tuned, detective we're far from finished cracking this case. Cue dramatic exit.

Gut Dysbiosis Disrupts Hair Health

Detective Detox was just getting comfortable after solving the toxin mystery when another case hit the desk. Reports were coming in: hair thinning, shedding, breakage hair crimes happening all over town. The victims? Innocent people just trying to live their best lives. The suspect? An internal mastermind wreaking havoc from within. Meet Dysbiosis, the shady character known for disrupting the balance of good and bad bacteria in the gut. And when Dysbiosis goes rogue, your hair follicles are often caught in the crossfire.

Join me as we dive deep into this tangled web of gut imbalance, nutrient theft, and inflammation, uncovering the role of gut dysbiosis in one of the most intricate hair sabotage schemes to date.

Imagine your gut as a bustling, harmonious city. In this city, there are good, hardworking citizens bacteria like Lactobacillus and Bifidobacterium who take care of everything, from digesting food to producing vitamins and fighting off invaders. But just like in any city, when things go wrong, chaos can ensue. The good bacteria get outnumbered by the bad guys harmful bacteria, yeasts, and fungi and before you know it, your once-thriving metropolis is in disarray. This is what we call gut dysbiosis.

When your gut microbiome a delicate ecosystem of trillions of microorganisms falls out of balance, it can have far-reaching consequences for your health, including, you guessed it, your hair. In this chapter, we'll delve into the world of gut dysbiosis, explore how an imbalanced microbiome affects your body, and most importantly, understand its impact on your hair. We'll also cover how to restore harmony in your gut to get your hair back to its crowning glory.

What Exactly is Gut Dysbiosis?

In a healthy gut, beneficial bacteria and other microorganisms work together to maintain balance. These good bacteria help digest food, produce essential nutrients like biotin and vitamin K, and keep the bad guys in check. But when the balance tips in favor of harmful bacteria, yeast, or fungi, gut dysbiosis occurs.

Gut dysbiosis can be triggered by several factors, such as:

- Poor diet (hello, processed foods and sugar!)
- Chronic stress (yes, that deadline at work isn't just bad for your sleep)
- Overuse of antibiotics (they don't just kill the bad bugs they wipe out the good guys too)
- Environmental toxins (from pesticides to pollution)
- Chronic illness (or simply feeling like you've been hit by a truck every day)

When dysbiosis strikes, it creates a domino effect in your body, causing inflammation, nutrient malabsorption, and you guessed it hair loss. But how does something happening in your gut lead to hair falling from your head? Let's find out.

The Gut-Hair Connection: When Chaos in the Gut Reaches the Scalp

Think of your hair follicles as delicate plants in a garden. They need nutrients, a balanced environment, and a lack of stress to thrive. But when your gut microbiome goes rogue, it's like turning the hose on full blast, pulling out the roots, and dumping junk in the soil. Here's how gut dysbiosis disrupts your hair health:

Inflammation: The Hair Follicle's Worst Nightmare

When harmful bacteria take over your gut, they trigger inflammation. These bad bacteria release toxins, which make their way into the bloodstream through the gut lining (especially if you have leaky gut syndrome, which we'll discuss soon). Once in your bloodstream, these toxins signal your immune system to go into overdrive.

Now, your immune system is amazing when it comes to fighting off infections, but it's a little too trigger-happy sometimes. The inflammation caused by these invaders doesn't just stay in your gut it travels everywhere, including to your hair follicles. And when hair follicles are inflamed, they can't function properly. This can lead to thinning hair, excess shedding, and in some cases, more severe hair loss conditions like alopecia areata.

Nutrient Absorption: Your Hair is Starving

Your hair needs essential nutrients to grow strong and healthy. Nutrients like biotin, zinc, iron, and B-vitamins are crucial for keeping those locks luscious. But when gut dysbiosis is present, your ability to absorb these nutrients becomes compromised.

Imagine you're at an all-you-can-eat buffet, but there's a bouncer at the door who won't let you in. That's essentially what's happening in your gut when dysbiosis is at play. The gut lining becomes inflamed, and the ability to absorb nutrients properly is significantly reduced. No matter how many leafy greens or biotin-packed foods you eat, your hair might not get the nutrients it needs, leading to weak, brittle hair or hair that simply doesn't grow as it should.

Hormonal Havoc: A Partnership in Crime

In case the nutrient theft and inflammation weren't enough, gut dysbiosis has another trick up its sleeve: hormonal sabotage. You've already met the key players in the hormone game estrogen, testosterone, and cortisol and you know they hold the power over your hair's fate. But did you know that gut dysbiosis can throw these hormones out of whack?

Here's how it works: your gut contains specific bacteria that help break down and metabolize hormones like estrogen. When the good bacteria are in charge, everything runs smoothly. Estrogen gets broken down and eliminated from the body efficiently. But when dysbiosis takes over, estrogen doesn't get cleared out it lingers in the bloodstream, leading to estrogen dominance. And as we know, too much estrogen is linked to hair thinning, especially in women.

But that's not all. Dysbiosis can also increase levels of cortisol, your body's main stress hormone. When cortisol levels stay high, it disrupts the hair growth cycle, pushing hair into the resting phase prematurely. And just like that, the hormonal balance is destroyed, and hair loss becomes the new normal.

Leaky Gut Syndrome: The Unwanted Guests

When dysbiosis persists, it can lead to something called leaky gut syndrome. Normally, your gut lining acts as a barrier, letting in only the nutrients you need and keeping harmful substances out. But when the gut lining becomes damaged, it's like someone punched holes in your city walls, allowing unwanted toxins, bacteria, and undigested food particles to leak into your bloodstream.

Now, imagine these toxins wandering around your bloodstream like uninvited guests at a party. Once they're loose in your system, they trigger even more inflammation and may lead to autoimmune responses where your body starts attacking itself including your hair follicles. This makes leaky gut syndrome one of the key culprits behind chronic hair loss conditions like alopecia.

So, what can you do to prevent dysbiosis from throwing your gut city into chaos and wreaking havoc on your hair? Let's explore ways to bring balance back.

What Causes Gut Dysbiosis?

While some causes of gut dysbiosis are out of your control (like genetics or chronic illness), many others are related to lifestyle choices. Here's what typically throws the gut out of whack:

1. Antibiotics: The Gut's Double-Edged Sword

While antibiotics are life-saving when it comes to fighting infections, they don't discriminate between the good bacteria and the bad. Think of antibiotics as a bomb that clears out all the residents of your gut city criminals and law-abiding citizens alike. This leaves the gut microbiome vulnerable, giving harmful bacteria the chance to take over. Frequent use of antibiotics without replenishing your good bacteria can lead to long-term dysbiosis.

2. Diet: Junk Food, Junk Gut

Your diet is one of the most significant factors influencing your gut microbiome. A diet high in processed foods, refined sugars, and unhealthy fats feeds harmful bacteria, allowing them to multiply and overpower beneficial bacteria. On the flip side, diets rich in fiber, prebiotics, and probiotics promote a healthy balance in the gut, which supports both digestion and hair growth.

3. Chronic Stress: Your Gut Feels It Too

Chronic stress doesn't just mess with your mind it messes with your gut too. The brain and gut are in constant communication via the gut-brain axis, and when you're stressed, your gut microbiome suffers. Stress leads to an increase in harmful bacteria, reduces beneficial bacteria, and contributes to inflammation, all of which lead to dysbiosis. So, yes, stressing out about your hair can actually make it worse!

4. Environmental Toxins: Hidden Saboteurs

We live in a world full of environmental toxins pollution, pesticides, plastics, and chemicals in household products. These toxins don't just affect your lungs or liver they disrupt your gut microbiome too. Exposure to these substances can alter your gut flora, reducing the diversity of beneficial bacteria and promoting the growth of harmful microbes.

Symptoms of Gut Dysbiosis

So, how do you know if your gut city has fallen into disarray? Here are some common symptoms of gut dysbiosis:

- **Digestive issues:** Bloating, gas, constipation, diarrhea, or a combination of these.
- **Chronic fatigue:** Feeling tired all the time, even after getting enough sleep.
- **Skin problems:** Acne, rashes, or eczema.
- **Brain fog:** Difficulty concentrating or remembering things.
- **Mood swings and anxiety:** A disrupted gut can influence your brain, leading to increased anxiety, irritability, or depression.
- **Weakened immune system:** Frequent colds or infections due to a weakened immune response.

And of course, one of the most telling symptoms hair thinning or loss. If you're experiencing one or more of these symptoms alongside changes in your hair, your gut might be trying to tell you something.

Healing Gut Dysbiosis for Hair Health

The good news is, gut dysbiosis doesn't have to be a permanent resident in your life. There are several steps you can take to restore balance to your gut microbiome and get your hair back on track. Think of it like performing a spring cleaning for your gut city, evicting the bad tenants and welcoming the good ones back.

1. Feed the Good Guys: Fiber and Prebiotics

Beneficial bacteria love to feed on prebiotics, which are indigestible fibers found in foods like garlic, onions, leeks, asparagus, and bananas. By incorporating more prebiotic-rich foods into your diet, you'll be supporting the growth of healthy bacteria and restoring balance in your gut. It's like giving your gut residents a feast!

In addition to prebiotics, aim for a diet rich in fiber, which promotes healthy digestion and keeps the gut moving. Whole grains, legumes, and vegetables are excellent sources of fiber that will help sweep out unwanted toxins and keep your gut functioning smoothly.

2. Repopulate with Probiotics

Once you've cleared out the harmful bacteria, it's time to invite the good ones back in. Probiotics are beneficial bacteria that help restore balance in the gut microbiome. You can find probiotics in fermented foods like yogurt, kefir, sauerkraut, kimchi, and kombucha. Or, if you prefer, you can take a high-quality probiotic supplement.

Probiotics help reduce inflammation, improve digestion, and enhance nutrient absorption all of which directly benefit hair growth. Think of them as the superheroes of your gut city, keeping the villains in check.

3. Avoid Sugar and Processed Foods

Harmful bacteria and yeast, like Candida, thrive on sugar. So, one of the best ways to starve out these bad guys is to reduce your intake of sugar and processed foods. This doesn't mean you have to swear off sweets forever, but cutting back on refined sugars, soft drinks, and junk food will help restore balance in your gut. Remember, every time you resist that candy bar, your hair thanks you!

4. Manage Stress

Since stress is a major trigger for gut dysbiosis, managing stress is essential for healing your gut and promoting hair growth. Incorporating stress-reduction practices like yoga, meditation, deep breathing, and regular exercise can help calm both your mind and your gut. And, let's be honest, your hair looks better when you're zen.

5. Stay Hydrated

Water is essential for keeping your digestive system moving and preventing constipation, which can worsen dysbiosis. Make sure you're drinking plenty of water throughout the day to support gut health and, ultimately, your hair. Think of hydration as the oil that keeps your gut's machinery running smoothly.

6. Consider Supplements

In some cases, specific supplements can help heal gut dysbiosis:

Probiotics:

As mentioned earlier, probiotics help repopulate the gut with beneficial bacteria. Look for a high-quality supplement with multiple strains of bacteria for the best results.

Digestive enzymes:

If your gut is struggling to break down food, digestive enzyme supplements can support proper digestion and nutrient absorption.

L-glutamine:

This amino acid helps heal the gut lining and reduce inflammation, making it a great option for those dealing with leaky gut syndrome.

Conclusion: Case Solved, Balance Restored

Detective Detox leans back in the chair, case file closed. Gut dysbiosis might be a sneaky villain, but we've cracked the case wide open. By restoring balance to the gut microbiome, we can stop dysbiosis in its tracks, reduce inflammation, and save your hair from its disastrous effects. The key is to bring in the good bacteria, feed them the right nutrients, and repair the gut barrier all while keeping stress levels in check.

Now that we've tackled this case, it's time to move on to the next chapter where we'll explore a more specific gut condition that's closely related to dysbiosis: leaky gut syndrome. We'll take a deep dive into how a leaky gut wreaks havoc on your health and hair and what you can do to seal the leaks and support both gut and hair health. But for now, rest easy knowing you've restored order to your gut, and your hair can finally start growing back stronger, thicker, and healthier. Cue detective music fade-out.

CHAPTER ELEVEN

Leaky Gut's Hair-Raising Consequences

Welcome to the world of Leaky Gut Syndrome a place where your gut, once a fortress of digestive fortitude, becomes more like a leaky sieve. Picture this: your gut lining, a strong security guard, standing at the border of your digestive system, carefully letting in only the best nutrients while keeping out the riff-raff. But when things go awry, it's as if your gut's security guard has taken an extended coffee break, letting in all the wrong elements bacteria, toxins, undigested food particles causing chaos throughout your body. And, of course, your hair is one of the first to feel the consequences.

In this chapter, we're diving into Leaky Gut Syndrome, a condition that not only makes you feel like your gut is staging a mutiny but also leads to hair loss, skin issues, fatigue, and general health mayhem. Don't worry there's hope. We'll talk about what causes leaky gut, how it sabotages your hair, and, most importantly, how to plug the leaks and get your body (and hair) back in shape.

What Is Leaky Gut Syndrome?
(And Why It Sounds Like a Plumbing Problem)

Leaky gut syndrome isn't a new designer diet, though it does sound trendy, doesn't it? "Leaky Gut: The Latest Hollywood Cleanse!" No, leaky gut happens when the intestinal lining normally a tight barrier that only let's essential nutrients through becomes too porous, allowing all sorts of unwelcome guests to slip through. Imagine your gut lining is like a carefully controlled club bouncer. Only the VIP nutrients get in, while toxins, undigested food particles, and bacteria are left outside.

But in leaky gut syndrome, that bouncer just throws open the doors and says, "Come on in, everyone!" And what happens next? Chaos. Toxins and bad bacteria flood into your bloodstream like uninvited guests at a party, wreaking havoc on your immune system, triggering inflammation, and making your hair go on strike.

How Does Leaky Gut Happen?

Great question! (Leaky Gut: not just for superheroes with digestive superpowers.) Several factors can cause the intestinal lining to become more permeable, including:

- **Poor diet** (aka too much processed junk food and sugar... hello, pizza, my old friend).
- **Chronic stress** (like when your mother-in-law comes over unannounced).
- **Overuse of antibiotics** (the nuclear option for gut bacteria good and bad).
- **Environmental toxins** (because we love spraying chemicals on things we eat).
- **Gut dysbiosis** (remember that gut city from Chapter 8 that turned into a bacterial Wild West?).

When these factors combine, they can damage the gut lining, creating little gaps that let toxins and undigested food particles leak into your bloodstream. It's like having a pickpocket in your gut, stealing your body's peace of mind and yes your hair.

What Happens When the Gut Leaks?

Here's where things get interesting (and a little messy). When those tiny cracks form in your intestinal wall, harmful substances like bacteria, toxins, and undigested food slip into your bloodstream, triggering the immune system to go into overdrive. It's like when your neighbor accidentally invites the local biker gang to their backyard barbecue, the immune system, much like an irritable neighbor, immediately overreacts.

This leads to chronic inflammation, which, as we've covered, is like kryptonite to your hair follicles. Chronic inflammation affects the entire body, including your scalp, where it can disrupt the hair growth cycle, making your hair thinner, weaker, and more likely to take a one-way trip down your shower drain.

Now, because this inflammation is happening in response to invaders (that shouldn't even be there in the first place), it's often linked to autoimmune conditions. This means your immune system, in its confused state, starts attacking your own body your joints, skin, and of course, your hair follicles.

How Leaky Gut Affects Hair Health

So, what does this mean for your hair? Spoiler alert: it's not good. Hair follicles are highly sensitive to changes in the internal environment, especially when it comes to inflammation and nutrient deficiencies. Leaky gut syndrome contributes to both, which results in the following hair-raising consequences:

1. Inflammation and Hair Loss: The Unwanted Duo

Inflammation is already a bad actor when it comes to hair health, but when your immune system is in full-blown attack mode thanks to toxins slipping through your gut, inflammation becomes a full-scale riot in your hair follicles. Chronic inflammation sends signals to the hair follicles to slow down the growth cycle. Hair goes from the anagen phase (growth) to the telogen phase (rest) faster than you can say, "Where did my hair go?"

In short, when your gut leaks, your immune system panics, inflammation rises, and your hair decides to check out of the growing business. The result? Thinning, shedding, and overall lackluster hair.

2. Nutrient Deficiencies: Your Hair's Famine

Your gut is responsible for absorbing nutrients from the food you eat, nutrients that are vital for hair growth like biotin, zinc, iron, and vitamins. But when your gut is leaking like an old garden hose, it's not absorbing those nutrients properly. No matter how many avocado toast breakfasts or spinach smoothies you consume, your body isn't getting the full benefit. Nutrient absorption becomes a mess, and your hair is left without the nourishment it needs to thrive.

Imagine trying to grow a lush garden without water or sunlight that's what's happening to your hair. It's malnourished, weak, and prone to breaking, and no amount of expensive hair serum can fix that.

3. Autoimmune Hair Loss: The Backstabbing Friend

Leaky gut is strongly linked to autoimmune conditions, where your immune system mistakenly attacks healthy cells. In the case of hair, this can lead to alopecia areata, a condition where the immune system attacks hair follicles, leading to patchy bald spots or, in more severe cases, total hair loss.

Alopecia is like that one friend who betrays you out of nowhere your immune system turns against your hair, creating bald spots, even though the hair itself isn't the problem. If you're experiencing patchy hair loss, leaky gut might be the root cause.

The Causes of Leaky Gut:
(Or How Your Gut Went From Bouncer to Party Animal)

So, how exactly did your gut lining become as porous as Swiss cheese? Here are the common causes of leaky gut syndrome:

1. Sugar: The Gut Villain

Sugar, while delicious, is like fertilizer for the bad bacteria in your gut. It feeds harmful microbes which can damage the gut lining and create those tiny cracks that lead to leaky gut. So, while that slice of cake might make you feel good for a minute, it's doing your gut and your hair no favors.

2. Processed Foods: Junk for the Gut, Junk for Your Hair

Processed foods are filled with preservatives, artificial colors, and unhealthy fats, all of which disrupt the gut microbiome and damage the gut lining. Plus, they're often low in fiber, which your good bacteria need to thrive. Think of processed foods as the fast-track to gut destruction.

3. Chronic Stress: The Gut's Frenemy

We know stress does horrible things to your gut (and your skin, and your mood, and your ability to avoid snapping at people...). Chronic stress increases cortisol, the stress hormone, which weakens the gut lining and increases gut permeability. Stress literally pokes holes in your gut, inviting toxins to wreak havoc.

4. Medications (Especially NSAIDs and Antibiotics)

While medications like antibiotics and NSAIDs (non-steroidal anti-inflammatory drugs) are useful when you need them, overuse can damage the gut lining and kill off beneficial bacteria, tipping the scales in favor of harmful microbes. Antibiotics are like gut bomb they wipe out everything, leaving your gut vulnerable and prone to leakage.

Symptoms of Leaky Gut (Aside from Bald Spots)

In addition to hair loss, leaky gut syndrome often comes with a host of other symptoms. If your gut is leaking like a faulty dam, you might experience:

- Bloating and gas (your jeans don't lie).
- Digestive issues (constipation or diarrhea, pick your poison).

- Brain fog (can't remember where you left your keys... or your car?).
- Fatigue (even after that fourth cup of coffee).
- Joint pain (creaky knees aren't just for grandpas anymore).
- Skin rashes (your gut and skin love to gossip about each other).

If these symptoms sound like you, it's time to investigate whether leaky gut syndrome is sabotaging your health and your hair.

How to Fix a Leaky Gut and Save Your Hair

Here's the good news: leaky gut isn't a life sentence. You can heal your gut lining, stop the leaking, and get your hair back on track with a few key lifestyle changes. Here's how to put your gut's bouncer back on duty and keep those toxins out:

1. Eliminate Gut-Damaging Foods

Start by removing the foods that are making your gut lining weaker. This includes:

Sugar (it's time to say goodbye, old friend).
Processed foods (that bag of chips is not your friend).
Gluten (for some people, gluten can increase gut permeability).
Dairy (if you're sensitive to lactose, it can also inflame the gut lining).

Replace these with whole, unprocessed foods that support gut health, like vegetables, lean proteins, and healthy fats.

2. Add Gut-Healing Foods

Your gut lining can repair itself with the right support. Foods that help heal the gut include:

Fermented foods: Sauerkraut, kimchi, kefir, and yogurt contain probiotics that restore balance to your gut microbiome.
Leafy greens: Packed with fiber, leafy greens feed the good bacteria in your gut, helping them thrive and keep the bad bacteria in check.

3. Take Gut-Healing Supplements

A few supplements can help speed up the process of healing leaky gut:

L-glutamine: This amino acid helps repair the gut lining, plugging up those leaks and preventing toxins from slipping through.
Probiotics: A high-quality probiotic can help restore balance to your gut flora and reduce inflammation.
Zinc: Zinc is crucial for maintaining the integrity of the gut lining. Plus, it's great for your skin and hair!

4. Reduce Stress

Stress might be a part of life, but chronic stress can wreck your gut. Incorporating stress-reducing activities like meditation, yoga, or even a daily morning walk can help reduce cortisol levels and support gut healing. Besides, your hair prefers you when you're calm.

5. Get Plenty of Sleep

Sleep is when your body does its repair work, and that includes fixing your gut. Aim for 6-8 hours of quality sleep each night to support gut healing and reduce inflammation. Early to bed and early to rise. Your hair will thank you!

Conclusion: Seal the Leaks, Save the Hair

Leaky gut syndrome might sound dramatic, but it's a fixable condition. By identifying and addressing the root causes whether it's stress, diet, or environmental factors you can heal your gut, reduce inflammation, and give your hair the support it needs to thrive.

In the next chapter, we'll dive into the power of probiotics and prebiotics for hair health and how you can harness the magic of these gut-boosting superstars to keep your hair strong and shiny from the inside out.

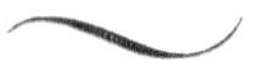

CHAPTER TWELVE

PROBIOTICS & PREBIOTICS - HAIR'S BEST FRIENDS

If someone told you that the secret to a thick, glossy mane wasn't in your bathroom cabinet but inside your gut, you'd probably give them the same look you reserve for people who suggest that pineapple belongs on pizza (because, let's be honest, the jury's still out on that one). But here's the thing: your gut is the backstage manager of your entire body, and if it's not doing its job properly, your hair's performance on the world stage is going to be a little... lackluster.

Enter the dynamic duo of probiotics and prebiotics the gut's very own superheroes. These little guys work behind the scenes to keep your gut (and, by extension, your hair) in tip-top shape. But first, let's clear something up: probiotics and prebiotics aren't the same thing. Probiotics are like the celebrity guests at your gut party, while prebiotics are the unsung heroes that make sure the catering is top-notch. Confused? Don't worry; by the end of this chapter, you'll be inviting both of these VIPs to every meal.

Let's get ready to rumble with the gut's power team, and maybe, just maybe, you'll have the best hair of your life while you're at it. Spoiler: this is one party your hair is going to love.

Probiotics: The Gut's A-List Celebrities

Probiotics are the rock stars of the gut microbiome. These beneficial bacteria are like your gut's personal army, defending against the bad guys (like harmful bacteria) and keeping everything running smoothly. They've got one job, and they're amazing at it: maintaining balance. And when your gut is balanced, your hair is more likely to flourish. You see, when probiotics are thriving in your digestive system, they keep inflammation down, nutrient absorption up, and your hair on your head where it belongs not circling the shower drain in a sad little pile.

But here's the kicker: your body doesn't naturally produce probiotics you have to invite them in. And just like inviting guests to a party, you need to be careful who you're bringing into your gut. You want the fun, responsible probiotics who'll make sure everyone has a good time, not the gatecrashers who spill drinks and start fights (we're looking at you, bad bacteria).

1. Where Do Probiotics Come From?

The best sources of probiotics come from fermented foods, which if you're not already familiar are foods that have been left out to develop their own beneficial bacteria (yes, it's weird science, but it works). These foods include:

Yogurt:
The OG of probiotics. Yogurt is packed with live cultures, especially if it's labeled with "live and active cultures." Just make sure you're avoiding the sugary, flavored varieties that sneak in more sugar than actual probiotics.
Kefir:
Think of kefir as yogurt's wild cousin. It's a fermented dairy drink with loads of probiotic bacteria that will make your gut (and hair) sing. If you can get past the weird sour tang, kefir is a winner.
Sauerkraut:
No, it's not just for your hotdog. Sauerkraut is basically cabbage that's been left to ferment its way into probiotic glory. Plus, it's loaded with fiber, making it a gut-loving powerhouse.

Kimchi:

This spicy Korean side dish is like sauerkraut on steroids. It's full of probiotics, and the spice gives it that extra kick, both for your taste buds and your gut health.

These foods are like the probiotic A-listers your gut needs to keep the party going, and the more diverse the probiotic strains, the better. It's like inviting guests from different backgrounds they bring a richer, more interesting vibe (and fewer awkward silences).

2. How Do Probiotics Help Your Hair?

By now, you might be wondering: "Sure, probiotics are great, but how does eating fermented cabbage or drinking sour milk help my hair?" Great question! Here's how:

Inflammation reduction:

Probiotics help reduce inflammation in the gut. And, as we've mentioned more times than your mother has reminded you to call her, inflammation is the enemy of hair follicles. When inflammation is under control, your hair follicles are less likely to throw in the towel and more likely to keep growing strong, healthy strands.

Nutrient absorption:

Probiotics help you absorb nutrients more efficiently. If your gut is doing a bad job at this (thanks to stress, poor diet, or letting the wrong bacteria run the show), it doesn't matter how many hair supplements you pop like candy your hair isn't getting the fuel it needs. Probiotics ensure that nutrients like biotin, zinc, and vitamin D actually make it to your hair follicles.

Scalp microbiome health:

Believe it or not, your scalp has its own microbiome (yep, more bacteria on your body!). Keeping your gut microbiome balanced can influence your scalp's health by reducing conditions like dandruff and scalp psoriasis, which contribute to hair thinning and loss.

In short, probiotics are like the bouncers at the door of your gut, making sure the VIPs (nutrients) get in while kicking out the rowdy troublemakers (bad bacteria) that want to mess with your hair's mojo.

Prebiotics: The Gut's Catering Service

Now, let's talk about prebiotics because even probiotics need a little help. Prebiotics are the food for probiotics. They're a type of fiber that humans can't digest but probiotics absolutely love. Think of prebiotics as the catering service at your gut's party without them, the probiotics don't have anything to munch on, and no party is fun when everyone's hangry.

The good news? You probably already eat prebiotics without realizing it. Foods like garlic, onions, bananas, and asparagus are packed with prebiotics. So, while you might think of onions as that smelly thing you chop up for dinner, to probiotics, it's a five-star meal.

1. Where Do Prebiotics Come From?

Prebiotics are found in various fiber-rich foods, including:

Garlic:
Turns out, garlic is not just great for scaring off vampires and annoying your date it's also packed with prebiotics that fuel your gut's beneficial bacteria.

Onions:
Another member of the smelly vegetable family that's secretly a gut superstar. Onions help your probiotics thrive, so don't skimp on them in your cooking (just maybe grab some breath mints).

Bananas:
When bananas get a little overripe, that's when they're loaded with prebiotics. So, the next time you see a spotty banana, don't throw it out your gut will thank you.

Asparagus:
Another sneaky prebiotic source. Asparagus doesn't just make your pee smell funny it's actually feeding the good bacteria in your gut and setting your hair up for success.

2. How Do Prebiotics Help Your Hair?

Without prebiotics, probiotics can't survive, and without probiotics, your gut microbiome becomes a disaster zone. Think of prebiotics as the secret sauce that keeps the whole operation running smoothly. Here's how prebiotics help your hair:

Fuel for probiotics: Prebiotics keep probiotics well-fed, which in turn keeps your gut in balance and your hair follicles healthy.
Fiber for digestion: Prebiotics are a type of fiber, and fiber is essential for keeping your digestion smooth. Smooth digestion means better nutrient absorption, which means stronger, shinier hair.

Basically, prebiotics are the unsung heroes of gut health. They're like that person who quietly does all the work at the office but never takes credit meanwhile, probiotics get all the praise. But we all know nothing would get done without prebiotics, and your hair wouldn't stand a chance without them.

The Probiotic-Prebiotic Power Couple: Gut Health's Dynamic Duo

When you combine probiotics and prebiotics, you've got the ultimate power couple for gut health. It's like pairing peanut butter with jelly, or if we're sticking with the party metaphor a DJ with the perfect playlist. One without the other just doesn't work as well. Together, they keep your gut microbiome balanced, inflammation in check, nutrient absorption optimized, and your hair in top form.

To really give your gut (and your hair) the star treatment, you need both probiotics and prebiotics in your diet. It's not enough to just chug kombucha and call it a day you've also got to feed those probiotics if you want them to stick around.

Probiotic Supplements: Gut Health in a Capsule

If fermented foods aren't your thing (or if the idea of eating sauerkraut every day gives you flashbacks to questionable high school lunches), don't worry probiotic supplements are here to save the day. These capsules contain live bacteria that make their way to your gut, ready to work their magic.

When choosing a probiotic supplement, it's important to look for a product with a variety of strains (because diversity is key!) and a high CFU count (that's colony-forming units basically, how many bacteria are in there). Look for a supplement with 10 billion CFUs or more, and bonus points if it has prebiotics mixed in.

How to Add Probiotics and Prebiotics to Your Routine (Without Going Overboard)

The great thing about probiotics and prebiotics is that you don't need to make massive changes to your diet to get their benefits. Here's how to add them to your daily routine without feeling like you've joined a weird food cult:

Start small:
You don't have to go full-on fermented right away. Try adding some yogurt or kefir to your breakfast or throwing a few fermented veggies on your salad.
Sneak in the prebiotics:
Toss some onions or garlic into your cooking (as if you weren't already!), and snack on bananas or apples for a prebiotic boost.
Mix and match:
Try to include a variety of probiotic and prebiotic foods throughout the week. It's all about diversity in your gut, so think of it like building a buffet for your bacteria.

Conclusion: Gut Health = Hair Health

At the end of the day, the key to great hair doesn't start with an expensive shampoo or fancy serum it starts in your gut. By nourishing your gut with the right balance of probiotics and prebiotics, you're giving your body the tools it needs to absorb nutrients, reduce inflammation, and keep your hair looking strong and vibrant.

In the next chapter, we'll dive into the lifestyle changes you can make to give your gut and hair the ultimate glow-up. From stress management to exercise and everything in between, get ready to transform your routine and unlock your hair's full potential.

CHAPTER THIRTEEN

THE GUT-HAIR ROUTINE

Congratulations, intrepid reader you've made it! You've journeyed through the winding roads of gut microbiomes, cortisol crises, probiotic superstars, yoga headstands, and even acupuncture needle therapy, all in the name of stronger, healthier hair. And now, here we are: the final chapter, where we tie it all together and create the ultimate gut-hair wellness routine that you can follow for life. This is your happy ending (complete with glorious, Instagram-worthy hair) because, let's face it, we all deserve to feel like a million bucks every time we look in the mirror.

Now, I know what you're thinking: "I've learned so much, but how do I actually make this work in my real life, where I still have work deadlines, laundry piles, and the occasional 3 AM existential crisis about whether or not I should've texted my ex?"

Fear not! This chapter is here to help you break it down, so you can implement these tips in the real world the one with busy schedules, imperfect days, and the occasional pizza night (because balance is everything). So grab your kombucha, fluff your hair, and let's dive into the Ultimate Gut-Hair Routine that will keep you smiling, stress-free, and with the kind of hair that makes strangers ask, "What's your secret?"

1. Morning Magic: Start Your Day Like You Mean It

Every successful routine begins with how you start your day. And I'm not talking about rolling out of bed, glaring at the alarm clock, and guzzling coffee like it's a life-saving elixir (though we've all been there).

I'm talking about creating a morning ritual that sets your gut and hair up for success from the moment you wake up. Because how you treat your body in the morning dictates how you'll feel and look for the rest of the day.

Your New Morning Game Plan:

Hydrate like a pro:
Start your day with a glass of warm water (with lemon, if you're feeling fancy). Your gut has been chilling overnight, and water helps wake it up, kickstarting your digestion and flushing out toxins. Plus, hydration is a hair lifesaver your hair is like a plant, and plants need water. Lots of it.

Probiotics before breakfast:
Whether it's a spoonful of yogurt or a probiotic supplement, getting some good bacteria into your system first thing in the morning gives your gut the boost it needs to function smoothly all day long. Bonus points if you pair it with a fiber-rich breakfast to feed your good gut buddies.

Mindful breathing or meditation:
Just 5–10 minutes of deep breathing or mindfulness meditation can set a peaceful tone for your day, keeping cortisol levels low and your gut stress-free. Your hair loves calm vibes. Trust me, this isn't just wellness mumbo jumbo it's science.
Less cortisol = less hair loss.

2. Feed Your Hair (and Gut) Throughout the Day

What you eat matters, but let's be clear this is not a call for perfection. You're not required to have spinach for every meal or suddenly turn into a salad person (unless you want to, in which case, salad cheers to you!). The goal here is balance: to give your gut the nutrients it needs to keep your hair strong while still enjoying life. Because hair health, much like everything else, thrives when you're happy and satisfied, not when you're obsessively counting calories or stressing over spinach and beetroot shortages at your local grocery store.

The Gut-Hair Power Plate:

Protein, please! Hair is made of keratin, which is a protein. If you're not getting enough protein, your hair will know and it will retaliate by becoming brittle and sad. Make sure every meal includes a good source of protein, like soyabeans, sprouts, pulses, eggs and chickpeas.

Fiber, fiber, fiber:
Your gut bacteria need fiber to thrive, and when your gut is happy, your hair is too. Load up on veggies, fruits, whole grains, and pulses to keep the good bacteria well-fed. Your hair will get all the nutrients it needs when your gut is doing its job.

Healthy fats for the win:
Omega-3 fatty acids are like the glitter of the nutritional world they make everything better. Found in pumpkin seeds, salmon, walnuts, chia seeds, and avocados, these healthy fats reduce inflammation, keep your scalp hydrated, and give your hair that enviable shine.

Snack smart:
Midday cravings happen, but instead of reaching for processed snacks that mess with your gut (and hair), grab gut-loving foods like carrots with hummus, a handful of almonds, or a probiotic-rich kombucha.

Watch the sugar:
Sugar feeds the bad bacteria in your gut, which leads to inflammation and as we know by now, inflammation is the villain in the hair story. Does this mean you can't have dessert? Of course not! Just don't let sugar steal the show from all the good things you're doing for your hair.

3. Move That Body, Boost That Hair

Exercise isn't just for your waistline or #fitspo posts on Instagram it's a secret weapon for both your gut and hairhealth. When you get your heart pumping, you boost circulation, which delivers oxygen and nutrients to your hair follicles. And let's not forget that exercise is the ultimate stress-buster, keeping those pesky cortisol levels at bay. The lower your stress, the more likely your hair will stay put on your head, where it belongs.

Exercise Hacks for Hair Health:

Daily movement:
Aim for at least 45 minutes of movement every day. This doesn't have to mean sweating it out in the gym (unless that's your thing). You can walk, dance in your living room, or do yoga in your PJs. Your gut and hair don't

care how you move just that you do.

Yoga for scalp circulation:

Incorporate yoga poses that promote blood flow to your scalp, like downward dog and forward folds. It's like sending a rush of nutrients directly to your hair follicles, and honestly, who doesn't want hair that feels as calm and flexible as they are?

Make it social:

Whether it's walking with a friend or joining a dance class, moving with others adds fun and accountability. And the laughter? That's just a bonus cortisol-lowering effect.

4. Stress Management: Chill for Better Hair

We've hammered this home by now, but it's worth saying one more time: stress is bad for your hair. Like, really bad. Stress triggers inflammation, messes with your gut, and kicks your hair into shedding mode faster than you can say, "I need a vacation." But managing stress doesn't mean you need to quit your job and move to a beach in Goa (though if you do, send me a postcard). It just means learning to handle stress in healthier ways, so your body and your hair don't take the hit.

Stress Management Superstars:

Meditation:

A repeat suggestion because it works. Just 10 minutes a day of sitting in stillness can lower cortisol and improve your gut health. Plus, your hair follicles get the message that it's okay to relax and keep growing.

Laughter:

Watch something funny, call up that friend who always makes you laugh, or scroll through memes. Laughter genuinely lowers stress hormones, so don't underestimate the power of a good giggle session for your hair's sake.

Gratitude journaling:

Studies show that gratitude reduces stress and boosts your mood. So, take a moment each day to jot down a few things you're thankful for. Bonus points if one of them is your fabulous hair-in-progress.

5. Sleep: The Ultimate Beauty Treatment

You've heard the term beauty sleep before, but it's not just a marketing gimmick. When you sleep, your body is in full-on repair mode, restoring your gut lining, reducing inflammation, and yes promoting hair growth. If you're skipping out on sleep, you're missing out on the most affordable (and effective) hair treatment ever. Plus, it feels amazing.

Sleep Essentials for Hair Health:

Set a bedtime routine:
Create a wind-down routine to signal to your body that it's time to relax. This could mean reading, sipping herbal tea, or dimming the lights and practicing some light stretching. Your gut, hair, and overall mood will benefit from a good night's sleep.

Get those 6-8 hours:
This isn't just a suggestion it's a non-negotiable. Your body needs that time to repair and refresh itself. Lack of sleep equals stressed-out hair follicles, so make sleep a priority.

Sleep on silk:
Want to get fancy? Switch to a silk pillowcase. Not only does it feel luxurious, but it also reduces friction on your hair, preventing breakage and keeping your strands smooth and tangle-free.

6. Pamper Your Scalp Like Royalty

Your scalp is the foundation of your hair's health. Think of it as the soil from which your hair grows. If the soil is dry, undernourished, or neglected, your hair won't thrive. So, treat your scalp like royalty it deserves it.

Scalp Care Rituals:

Weekly scalp massages:
Massaging your scalp with a nourishing oil (like coconut or rosemary oil) not only feels heavenly but also promotes blood flow to the hair follicles, encouraging growth. Plus, it's a stress-relieving ritual in itself.

Exfoliate your scalp:
Just like your skin, your scalp needs exfoliation to remove dead skin cells

and product buildup. Use a gentle scalp scrub once a week to keep your scalp clean and your hair follicles happy.

Keep it clean, but not too clean:
Washing your hair regularly is important, but over-washing can strip your scalp of natural oils. Aim for 2-3 washes a week, depending on your hair type, and use a gentle shampoo that doesn't disrupt your scalp's microbiome.

Conclusion: Own Your Gut, Love Your Hair, Live Your Best Life

You've done it. You've completed the Ultimate Gut-Hair Wellness Routine, and you are now armed with all the knowledge (and humor) you need to take control of your gut, love your hair, and live your best life. The key takeaway? It's all connected. Your gut, your stress levels, your diet, your sleep it all comes together to create the perfect environment for healthy, vibrant hair.

Remember, this isn't about perfection. You don't have to do every single thing every day, but making small, consistent changes will have a big impact over time. When you take care of your gut, you're not just helping your hair you're improving your overall well-being. And that, my friend, is worth every green smoothie, scalp massage, and mindful breath.

So go ahead, flaunt that hair, smile with confidence, and know that you've unlocked the secret to thriving from the inside out. Here's to a life of happy gut, fabulous hair, and endless good vibes. Now, go live your best, most radiant self!

Next in line is something new and interesting .. stay tuned !!

CHAPTER FOURTEEN

BIOHACKING FOR GUT AND OPTIMAL HAIR

A New Dawn: The Rise of Biohacking

Imagine a world where you have the tools, knowledge, and technology to become your own health expert a world where you are empowered to understand how your body works and make precise changes to optimize every aspect of your well-being, from your digestion to your hair growth. Welcome to the world of biohacking.

Biohacking is all about taking control of your own biology. It's the art and science of using personalized strategies, from diet and lifestyle changes to advanced technologies, to enhance your body's performance and optimize health. And when it comes to hair health, biohacking offers an innovative approach to improving your gut microbiome, balancing your hormones, and creating an environment where your hair can grow stronger, shinier, and fuller than ever before.

In this chapter, we'll dive into the exciting world of biohacking what it is, how it works, and, most importantly, how you can use it to transform your gut and hair health.

Biohacking Basics: The Key Principles

Before diving into the specific techniques and strategies for hair health, let's outline the key principles of biohacking. By understanding these foundational concepts, you'll be equipped to make more informed decisions and customize your approach to suit your unique needs.

Self-Experimentation and Data Tracking

One of the core principles of biohacking is self-experimentation trying out different strategies, tracking how your body responds, and making adjustments based on your observations. This is where data tracking comes in. By collecting information about your diet, lifestyle, sleep, stress levels, gut health, and hair growth, you can identify patterns, discover what works best for you, and make targeted changes.

Personalization – One Size Doesn't Fit All

Biohacking recognizes that everyone's biology is different, and what works for one person may not work for another. Genetics, lifestyle, diet, and environment all play a role in shaping how your body functions. The goal of biohacking is to find what works for *you* customizing your approach to align with your unique needs and goals. Personalization means experimenting with different foods, supplements, and lifestyle habits to see what makes u feel and look best. U need to approach it with curiosity and an open mind, knowing that there may be some trial and error along the way.

Root Cause Resolution – Not Just Symptom Management

Biohacking is about addressing the root causes of health issues, not just managing symptoms. When it comes to hair loss, this means going beyond topical treatments and quick fixes to explore the underlying factors that contribute to poor hair health, such as nutrient deficiencies, hormonal imbalances, stress, and gut dysbiosis. By focusing on root causes, u can make lasting changes that not only improve your hair growth but also enhance your overall health, energy levels, and well-being.

The Biohacking Toolkit: Strategies for Gut and Hair Health

Now that we've covered the basics, let's dive into the biohacking toolkit an arsenal of strategies, tools, and techniques that you can use to optimize your gut microbiome and hair health. Each tool is designed to target a specific aspect of health, and when used together, they create a holistic approach to improving hair growth from the inside out.

Tool #1: Microbiome Testing – Mapping the Gut

If the gut is the foundation of hair health, then understanding the state of your gut microbiome is essential. One of the first biohacks to try is microbiome testing, a process that involves analyzing the bacteria in your gut to determine its composition, diversity, and overall balance. Microbiome testing can reveal the presence of beneficial bacteria, harmful pathogens, and potential dysbiosis (imbalance in the gut microbiome).

You can use a home testing kit that requires a stool sample, which then needs to be sent to a lab for analysis. The results provide a detailed report of your gut bacteria, as well as personalized recommendations for improving your microbiome.

With this knowledge, you can make targeted changes to your diet and lifestyle to promote the growth of these beneficial bacteria, such as adding more fermented foods, prebiotic fibers, and probiotic supplements to your routine.

Tool #2: Intermittent Fasting – Resetting the Body's Rhythm

Intermittent fasting (IF) is a biohacking practice that involves cycling between periods of eating and fasting. While fasting may seem daunting at first, it can have numerous health benefits, including improving gut health, enhancing nutrient absorption, reducing inflammation, and promoting hormonal balance all of which support healthy hair growth.

You can decide decides to try a 16:8 or a 12:12 intermittent fasting schedule, where one fasts for 16 hours and has an 8-hour eating window or fast for 12 hours and have a 12 hour eating window. The fasting period allows the gut to rest, repair, and reset, and you can notice improved digestion, increased energy levels, and reduced sugar cravings over time.

While IF may not be suitable for everyone, you can find that it helps to develop a more mindful approach to eating and creates a positive ripple effect on your gut and hair health.

Tool #3: Adaptogens – Balancing Stress and Hormones

Adaptogens are natural herbs and plants that help the body adapt to stress, balance hormones, and support overall resilience. Since chronic stress is a major contributor to gut imbalance and hair loss, you can incorporate adaptogens into your daily routine as part of your biohacking strategy.

Some of the adaptogens you can experiment with include:

- **Ashwagandha**: A calming adaptogen that helps reduce cortisol levels and improve sleep quality.
- **Rhodiola Rosea**: Known for boosting energy, mental focus, and resilience to stress.
- **Holy Basil (Tulsi)**: Helps balance blood sugar levels and reduce anxiety, supporting a calm and focused state of mind.

You can start by adding ashwagandha to your evening routine, either in the form of a supplement or as a powder mixed into warm almond milk. Over time, you can notice a significant reduction in stress, better sleep, and more balanced energy levels creating an environment where your hair can grow more effectively.

Tool #4: Red Light Therapy – Boosting Hair Growth with Light

One of the most fascinating biohacks that can be tried is red light therapy, also known as low-level laser therapy (LLLT). Red light therapy involves exposing the scalp to low-level red or near-infrared light, which has been shown to stimulate hair follicles, improve blood circulation, and promote hair growth.

You can use a red light therapy device that can be worn on your head for 10-20 minutes a day. The light penetrates the scalp, increasing cellular activity in the hair follicles and boosting collagen production, which is essential for hair strength and elasticity. This biohack is non-invasive, safe, and easy to incorporate into you daily routine whether you are working, relaxing, or reading a book.

Over time, you may notice that the hair feels thicker, shinier, and less prone to breakage. Red light therapy, combined with other biohacks, may create a multi-dimensional approach to supporting hair health.

Tool #5: Bulletproof Coffee and MCT Oil – Fueling the Brain and Gut

One of the staples of the biohacking world is "Bulletproof Coffee" a blend of coffee, MCT oil (medium-chain triglyceride oil), and grass-fed butter or ghee. While it might sound unusual, this concoction is designed to provide sustained energy, mental clarity, and support for gut health.

MCT oil, in particular, is a biohacker's secret weapon. It's a type of fat that is easily absorbed by the body and provides quick energy to both the brain and gut. MCT oil also has antimicrobial properties, which can help balance the gut microbiome and promote digestion.

You can start mornings with Bulletproof Coffee, and that it keeps you full, energized, and focused for hours. It also provides healthy fats that support hormone balance and nourish your hair follicles from within.

Tool #6: Cold Therapy – Boosting Circulation and Reducing Inflammation

Cold therapy, also known as cryotherapy, is another biohacking technique that can improve hair health by boosting circulation, reducing inflammation, and stimulating the scalp. Cold therapy can be as simple as taking a cold shower, using an ice roller on the scalp, or immersing the body in cold water (like a cold plunge or ice bath).

While the idea of cold showers may sound daunting, once can decide to try it out for the benefits it offers. You can start with contrast showers alternating between hot and cold water for a few minutes each day. The cold water stimulates blood flow to the scalp, delivering oxygen and nutrients to hair follicles while reducing inflammation.

You might find that while the first few seconds are intense, your body with quickly adapts to the cold and feels invigorated afterward. Over time, your hair may appears fuller, and experience less scalp irritation and inflammation.

The Art of Biohacking: Making It Your Own

Biohacking isn't a one-size-fits-all solution it's about experimenting, tracking progress, and making adjustments based on what works best for you. As you explore the world of biohacking, remember that the goal is to make it fun, enjoyable, and aligned with your unique needs. Whether you choose to try microbiome testing, intermittent fasting, adaptogens, red light therapy, Bulletproof Coffee, or cold therapy, the key is to listen to your body, track your progress, and make adjustments along the way.

Biohacking is about becoming the architect of your health, empowering yourself to make informed decisions that support not only your hair but your overall well-being. It's a journey of exploration, self-care, and optimization a journey where you are both the conductor and the musician of your own life's symphony.

So go ahead experiment, discover, and unlock your optimal hair potential. Your gut, hormones, and hair follicles are ready to thrive.

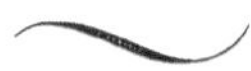

Conclusion: Gut-brain-hair Connection

And here we are, at the glorious finale of your journey through the fascinating, often unexpected, and deeply intertwined world of the gut-brain-hair axis. If you've made it this far, you've done more than just read a book you've taken a transformative step toward owning your wellness, understanding your body's intricate systems, and empowering yourself to live healthier, happier, and, let's not forget, more fabulous hair days.

Throughout this journey, you've discovered that hair health isn't just about shampoos and serums. Your hair is a reflection of everything going on beneath the surface, your gut health, your stress levels, the nutrients you take in, and even the way you sleep and move. It's a complex, symphonic relationship where every part of your body plays a key role, and like any good conductor, you're now fully equipped to orchestrate your health from the inside out.

You Hold the Power

The true power of this book lies in one simple idea: you hold the key to your body's well-being. No one else. Not your hairstylist, not the latest hair-care brand, not even that trendy wellness guru on social media. It's you, your habits, your choices, and your ability to listen to your body and nurture it in ways that work for you.

You've learned that gut health is the foundation of your entire body's well-being, and by nurturing it, you're setting the stage for strong, vibrant hair. But beyond hair, you're also nourishing your brain, your immune system, your digestion, and even your mental health. It's a holistic approach that doesn't just change your reflection in the mirror it changes how you feel in your skin, every day.

A Lifestyle, Not a Fad

Unlike the countless quick-fix solutions out there, what you've discovered in this book is a lifestyle change one that's sustainable, realistic, and designed to bring out the best in you. It's not about overnight transformations or unrealistic expectations. It's about long-term wellness, and understanding that the body and mind thrive on balance and care, not punishment and stress.

The magic of this journey is that it's not just about hair. Yes, you'll enjoy healthier, thicker, and shinier locks, but you'll also experience a ripple effect in every aspect of your life. More energy, better mood, deeper sleep, and improved resilience to stress these are the ultimate rewards when you start healing from within.

You've Got This

Life will always throw challenges your way whether it's a stressful work week, a busy family schedule, or the temptation of convenience food when you're just too tired to cook. But now you know how to tackle these challenges. You've learned that taking care of yourself isn't selfish it's necessary. And you've discovered that small, consistent changes can lead to big results.

Remember, this isn't about perfection. There will be days when you miss your yoga class or forget to take your probiotics. That's okay! What matters is the overall journey your commitment to yourself and your well-being. Your hair, your body, and your mind will thank you for the effort, even on the imperfect days.

The Gut-Brain-Hair Connection: A New Way of Living

As you close this book, know that you've gained far more than just knowledge about hair health. You've tapped into the deeper wisdom of your body the way it communicates, heals, and grows. You've embraced the gut-brain-hair connection, which isn't just a wellness concept it's a roadmap to living your best life.

So, let this be the beginning of your new journey one where you approach health not as a chore but as a celebration. Where you listen to your gut, nurture your body, and honor your mind. And most importantly, where you embrace your inner and outer beauty with the confidence and power you deserve.

Your hair is your crown, and you now have the knowledge to wear it proudly healthy, strong, and shining from the inside out. You've started a revolution in your body, a revolution of self-care, balance, and true wellness.

Now go out there and rock that crown. Your best hair and your best self await.

Thank you for joining this journey. Here's to your thriving gut, your glowing hair, and your beautifully empowered life!